Inclusion

Including People With Disabilities in Parks and Recreation Opportunities

Inclusion

Including People With Disabilities in Parks and Recreation Opportunities

Lynn Anderson, PhD, CTRS
and
Carla Brown Kress, MEd, CTRS

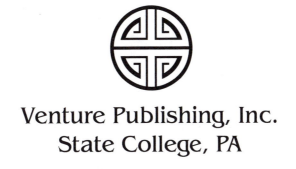

Venture Publishing, Inc.
State College, PA

Venture Publishing, Inc.
1999 Cato Avenue
State College, PA 16801
Phone: (814) 234–4561
Fax: (814) 234–1651

Production Manager: Richard Yocum
Manuscript Editing: Valerie Paukovits, Richard Yocum
Cover Design: Echelon Design
Cover Photograph: Corbis

Unless otherwise noted, photographs courtesy of Lynn Anderson or Carla Brown Kress

Library of Congress Catalogue Card Number 2003101466
ISBN 1–892132–33–8

Table of Contents

Staff
Marketing
Traits of a Quality Program
Assignment: Equal Opportunity Recreation Provider

Acknowledgments

This book was originally developed as a training manual for the Rural Recreation Integration Project, a grant project funded by the U.S. Department of Education, Office of Special Education and Rehabilitative Services. We would like to thank Patricia Soli for her invaluable work with the grant project and the extensive training and technical assistance it entailed. We would also like to acknowledge the North Dakota Department of Parks and Recreation for its vision and support of inclusion of people with disabilities in parks and recreation through its active involvement in the grant project. Instrumental in the project was Tim Mueller, formerly with the department. We would like to thank the numerous Rural Recreation Integration Project participants with whom this book was field-tested—professionals in parks, recreation, and human services; parents of children with disabilities; adults with disabilities; self-advocates; and others. Though they deserve acknowledgment for their successful efforts in making inclusion happen, they are too numerous to mention by name.

This manual grew out of the work of the grant project, with numerous reiterations as it was used in training over a 3-year period. It is based on a strong foundation learned from experts in the area of inclusion and recreation. We would like to acknowledge and thank them for their continuing advancement of our knowledge base in this area. In particular, we would like to thank Dr. Stuart Schleien, Dr. Linda Heyne, Dr. Carol Stensrud, Cynthia Burkhour, and Dr. John Dattilo.

We would also like to acknowledge our respective employers—the Eden Prairie, Minnesota Parks, Recreation, and Natural Resource Department and the State University of New York at Cortland—for their support of our work in inclusion and recreation and their belief in its importance. In addition, we would like to thank Richard Yocum and Valerie Paukovits of the Venture Publishing editorial staff for their support and guidance in bringing this book to fruition.

Lastly, we would like to thank our supportive families: Dale, Kelly, and Cory Anderson and Darren, Zach, and Sam Kress.

Foreword

I am honored to introduce this excellent book on inclusion that Dr. Lynn Anderson and Carla Brown Kress have so thoughtfully written. For those of us who seek to realize the dream of inclusive community leisure services, this text serves as an exceptional resource for educating others about inclusion and how to make this ideal a working reality.

Inclusion: Including People With Disabilities in Parks and Recreation Opportunities grew from a training manual developed through the Rural Recreation Integration Project, a 3-year federally funded project in North Dakota spearheaded by the authors and Patricia Soli. I was excited when Dr. Anderson asked me to become involved in the project by facilitating focus groups around the state to assess opinions about inclusion and to determine what training would be needed to promote inclusive programming.

The training manual ultimately developed from this project was an outstanding resource on inclusion presented in a format that readily engaged the reader. Many times as I prepared to teach a class or an in-service on inclusion, I went to my bookshelf and reached for this manual. I often recommended the manual to others, though I forewarned that its availability was limited. It is wonderful that Venture Publishing has taken up the publication of this material so it is now more widely available to a larger audience.

While traveling the highways of North Dakota with Dr. Anderson and Ms. Brown conducting focus groups, I not only experienced unexpected winter whiteouts and beautiful prairie sunsets, but also came to know the authors and their tireless commitment to inclusion much better. It is their commitment to inclusion—their dedication, openness, enthusiasm, perseverance, and creativity—evident in their first manual that now permeates this entire book.

This volume gets at the heart of inclusion in a way both comprehensive and direct. All the key issues related to inclusion are addressed—the philosophical premises, physical and programmatic accessibility, administrative concerns (e.g., staffing and safety), networking, and how to overcome obstacles (e.g., attitudinal and architectural barriers). Further, as much as I appreciate *what* the book says, I appreciate *how* the authors have chosen to say it. Each chapter is logically and clearly organized. Key messages are delivered clearly and powerfully. Assignments and sample scenarios encourage the reader to actively grapple with the questions that inclusion raises in a personal and thought-provoking way.

The overall effect of this book is one that communicates the power of education to change society. Whether you are a parent, self-advocate, therapeutic recreation specialist, leisure services practitioner, human services professional, student, or professor, you will find this book useful in educating yourself and others about inclusion. The conceptual and practical information contained in this book will inspire the reader to take initiative to support inclusion of individuals with disabilities in the life of their communities. I wish to thank the authors for offering such a valuable, usable, and insightful addition to the inclusion literature.

Linda A. Heyne, PhD, CTRS
Ithaca College
Ithaca, New York

Introduction: About This Manual

People with disabilities now reside primarily in community settings. This has not always been the case. Less than 20 years ago many people with disabilities lived in institutional settings, such as state hospitals, state schools, and nursing homes. As society's attitude toward people with disabilities changed, and as legislation changed, more people moved into our communities to less restrictive environments. Although communities have been able to provide housing and some human and education services, many people with disabilities are not yet a part of the fabric of communities.

The Rural Recreation Integration Project, a 3-year grant project funded by the U.S. Department of Education, Office of Special Education and Rehabilitative Services, had as its vision the inclusion of people with disabilities in the fabric of community life. This manual grew out of the training provided by the Rural Recreation Integration Project, a collaborative effort between the North Dakota Parks and Recreation Department and the University of North Dakota. The Rural Recreation Integration Project worked to bridge the gap between two service delivery systems: recreation and leisure services and human services. It intended to develop naturally sustaining networks where resources and expertise could be shared to most effectively meet the recreation needs of people with disabilities in their communities. People with disabilities or their advocates and families have expertise in disability and are aware of the leisure and social needs and barriers they face. Professionals in human services come in contact with people with disabilities on a regular basis. Recreation and leisure service providers have the facilities, resources, and expertise in recreation programming, but may lack awareness of the needs of people with disabilities living in their communities or how to meet them. By bringing these professionals together, providing training and technical assistance, and involving people with disabilities, inclusive recreation services become a reality. (See Appendix A for more information on the Rural Recreation Integration Project.)

The purpose of this manual is to provide information and resources for professionals in parks and recreation and human services to facilitate inclusive recreation services. The manual presents clear strategies to include people with disabilities in community recreation opportunities. It is based on the belief that inclusion happens one person at a time, and that each person participating in recreation programs, including a person with a disability, is a unique individual with unique needs.

Each chapter is laid out in a format that could easily be used in staff training sessions. In addition to the main content, each chapter ends with an interactive assignment that either clarifies the concepts in the chapter or helps readers to put the material into practice in their agencies.

Chapter 1 provides a foundation to the remaining chapters by exploring and clarifying the concepts of recreation and leisure. A clear understanding of the critical elements of quality recreation and leisure will facilitate inclusion of people with disabilities in those experiences. This conceptual foundation will help to prevent common pitfalls often encountered in providing recreation experiences to people with disabilities, such as stereotyped activities (e.g., bowling, Special Olympics) or the provision of convenient activities to "keep 'em busy." Every person's interests in recreation must be fostered to bring quality to his or her life.

Chapter 2 overviews the concept of inclusion and its benefits to participants with and without disabilities. This chapter presents the concept of person-first language and the importance of our attitudes in promoting inclusive leisure services.

Chapter 3 provides a comprehensive framework for understanding physical accessibility and how to assess your agency and facilities for accessibility. The Americans with Disabilities Act is presented, along with accessibility standards that provide

People with disabilities are physically included in our communities, but not necessarily socially included.

Inclusion works best when networks of people with disabilities, human service providers, and recreation professionals all work together.

Inclusion happens one person at a time.

accessible environments. Suggestions for improving accessibility for various types of disabilities are provided.

Making a building or area physically accessible is only a small part of inclusion, however. *Chapter 4* provides a clear process to understand and to implement programmatic, or social, inclusion. Each step of the process is discussed, and a case study is provided that illustrates the whole process in an actual recreation setting. Staff training, an important step in the inclusion process, is focused on in depth, and the chapter provides assignments that can be used in staff training.

Chapter 5 addresses important administrative concerns with inclusion, from mission and philosophy to funding and liability. Without administrative support, inclusion will not prosper at any agency. This chapter provides information to help inclusion happen from the top down and to complement efforts at the individual and program level.

Chapter 6 focuses in-depth on networking, a critical aspect of successful inclusion efforts. Because no one agency has all the resources, expertise, or access to participants to fully implement inclusion, networking becomes essential in pooling energy and talent to facilitate leisure experiences for all. This chapter shares model programs as a way to illustrate the importance of networking and to provide important role models and contacts for others as they begin to develop inclusion efforts at their agencies.

Because challenges exist when change is implemented, *Chapter 7* overviews some of the challenges commonly experienced as agencies work toward inclusion, as well as some strategies to handle those challenges more effectively.

The *Appendices* provide valuable resources for the reader. Because we believe that inclusion is best facilitated by focusing on the person and not the disability, we put disability-related information at the end of the book . Also in the appendices are sample staff training exercises and job descriptions, as well as sample forms for intake, assessment, program documentation, and evaluation. It is our hope that these useful tools can be adapted and easily used to help the reader more easily put inclusion into practice.

Lastly, the *References and Resources* section allows the reader to get more in-depth information on the concepts and materials presented in the book.

Overall, this book intends to serve as a tool to facilitate inclusion in the everyday world of recreation program delivery. Although it focuses on disability, the concepts and processes can be used to facilitate inclusion of all people with differences. We would like to see it used at the practitioner level as a staff training manual and as a reference accessed on a daily basis as inclusion is implemented in programs and facilities. Feedback on its usefulness would be greatly appreciated by the authors.

If the only tool you have is a hammer, you tend to see every problem as a nail.
—Abraham Maslow

Chapter 1

Why Is Recreation Important to People With Disabilities?

Why are recreation, play, and leisure important for people with disabilities? To answer this question, one must ask, "Why are recreation and leisure important to me?" Many people, whether they have a disability or not, do not stop to seriously think about the importance of recreation and leisure in their lives. It is an area often taken for granted and thought of as less important than work. Many people with a very strong work ethic may view leisure, play, and recreation as wasteful, childish, and unimportant.

To the contrary, leisure plays a very important role in our lives and helps to shape who we are as human beings. When people are not allowed opportunities for play, recreation, and leisure it affects their physical, intellectual, social, and emotional development and well-being. (Before proceeding, complete the assignment on p. 6.)

Leisure helps to shape who we are as human beings.
—Russell

Leisure: Three Common Meanings

Leisure as Free Time

Leisure can be considered time free from obligations—time at one's disposal. To some people, leisure is the weekend (Russell, 2002).

What does leisure mean to you?

Leisure as Recreational Activity

Leisure can be considered nonwork activity, such as sports, games, art, music, hobbies, rest, and social interaction. The activity is freely chosen and benefits the individual.

Leisure as Attitude

Leisure can be considered how one feels about the activity being pursued or the time being spent. It is feelings of self-satisfaction, positive outlook, and happiness. Leisure provides opportunities for self-expression, self-achievement, and self-actualization.

Recreation Is...

Recreation is commonly defined as activities developed by society for the primary reasons of fun and enjoyment. Recreation refers to the activity itself and is independent of how one feels about participation in that activity. Recreation includes activities that society feels are positive and contribute to individual and societal well-being. Often recreation is thought of as sports and other activities organized by a group, such as a park district or YMCA. It is important to remember that recreation includes not only sports, but also a wide array of positive free time activities, from cultural activities to entertainment to intellectual activities.

Recreation
Organized activities for fun and enjoyment that society feels are positive

Play Is...

Play is the spirit of leisure.

Play is the spirit of leisure. It is spontaneous, carefree, imaginative, and creative. Play is not for the sake of a final goal—it is motivated by the enjoyment of living. Play, though most often associated with children, is important in all human activity across the life span. It is through play that humans experience joy, zest, and self-expression. All people need to play to experience quality of life.

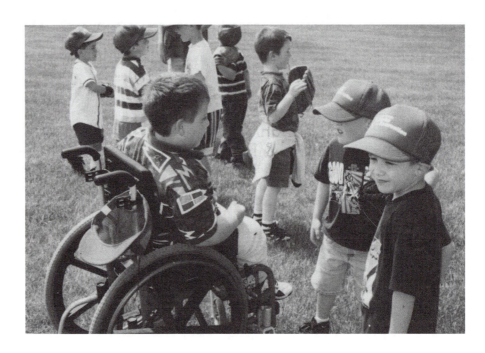

I can learn more about a person in an hour of play than in a lifetime of conversation.
—Plato

Qualities That Make Experiences Leisure, Recreation, or Play

Leisure has the greatest potential of all human arenas to produce boredom—it must be quality leisure to be pleasurable and personally meaningful.
—Russell

Free time or nonwork activities are not necessarily rewarding and fulfilling. Leisure has the greatest potential of all human arenas to produce boredom (Russell, 2002). "Filling up a person's time" or "keeping busy" do not ensure high quality leisure. For leisure to be pleasurable and personally meaningful, it must be quality leisure. The following list includes qualities that make experiences truly *leisure* experiences.

Freedom

People need to have a sense of freedom to make the choices they want for their leisure, as opposed to being pressured into a certain choice.

Choice

People need an array of opportunities available to them for leisure experiences.

Internal Rewards

People need to do leisure activities because of how they will feel inside—the positive feelings and benefits derived from involvement in the leisure experience. People do not choose leisure for trophies, praise, or other external rewards.

Sense of Control

People need to feel a sense of control during a leisure experience—a sense that they can positively control the outcomes of the experience.

Optimal Arousal

Quality leisure experiences make people sharply aware of and in tune with their surroundings and the activity. They feel "really alive" and time flies by.

Novelty

Leisure experiences need to be different from the normal routine of people's lives.

Challenge

People need to feel that they are using their skills and abilities and exerting effort (physical, social, intellectual, or emotional) during the leisure experience.

What Are the Benefits of Leisure and Recreation?

Much research documents the benefits of leisure, play, and recreation (Canadian Parks/Recreation Association, 1997; Parks and Recreation Federation of Ontario, 1992). These benefits range from personal to social to economic to environmental. The benefits that can be received from leisure are important to all people, with and without disabilities.

What Are Some *Personal* Benefits of Leisure and Recreation?

- Recreation contributes greatly to a full and meaningful life—a life worth living.

- Regular physical activity is one of the best ways to assure good physical and mental health.

- Leisure helps to manage stress in a busy world.

- Leisure meaningful to us helps to increase self-esteem and to promote good feelings about ourselves and our lives.

- Leisure helps us to to lead balanced and full lives, to achieve our full potential, and to gain life satisfaction.

- Leisure provides positive lifestyle choices and alternatives to self-destructive behavior.

- Leisure and play are essential to the human development process. Many skills necessary for successful participation in other aspects of life are learned during leisure.

- People gain satisfaction and a higher quality of life when they can recreate in parks, open spaces, and other aesthetic and diverse environments.

I ride the city bus around for fun. There's not much else for me to do, because I don't like sports and that's all they have for people like me.
—Ellen, a 64-year-old woman with mental retardation

Leisure and recreation offer both personal and social benefits.

People do not cease to play because they grow old; they grow old because they cease to play.
—George Bernard Shaw

What Are Some *Social* Benefits of Leisure and Recreation?

- Leisure provides opportunities to build stronger communities.

- Recreation reduces alienation, loneliness, and antisocial behaviors.

- Community recreation promotes diversity and increased understanding of differences between people.

- Recreation builds strong families.

- Leisure provides opportunities for community involvement and friendship development.

- Community pride is higher when quality recreation opportunities are available for all people.

Leisure and recreation are important for people with disabilities for the same reasons they are important to all people. However, due to limited opportunities to participate fully in recreation and leisure, people with disabilities have not always been able to realize the same benefits. It is important for our society to learn how to provide recreation and leisure opportunities that are inclusive and open to *all* people.

If one has limited opportunities for recreation and leisure, one will realize only limited benefits.

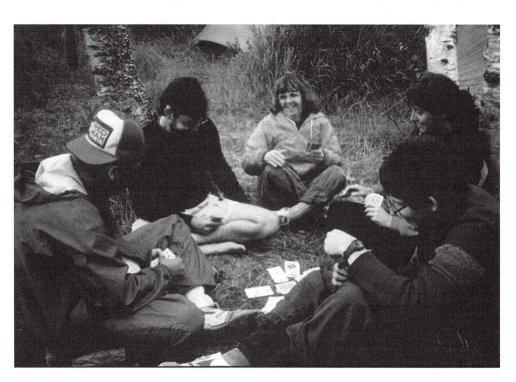

Everyone's Leisure and Recreation Interests Are Different

When planning recreation and leisure opportunities, remember that everyone's interests are different. One historical way of providing recreation services for people with disabilities was to provide segregated activities that offered few choices. Bowling and "handicapped gym" are two examples of commonly offered segregated activities. It is imperative that people with disabilities be asked what they like and want for leisure and not be offered only special needs programs that have little to do with their interest areas.

Get to know the needs and interests of participants—do not assume.

People With Disabilities May Have Less Experience With Leisure

Research has shown that people with disabilities participate less in all forms of recreation than other individuals, but may have more free time. Due to a lack of exposure, lack of opportunities, overreliance on segregated programs, and negative attitudes, some people with disabilities may need help discovering their interests, while others may want to explore new leisure interests. Determine an individual's preferences, then help him or her to gain access and skills in those activities.

While leisure is assumed to be an important aspect in the quality of life for all people, those with disabilities are often unable to take full advantage of the potential for leisure in their lives. This must be changed, because leisure provides opportunities for freedom, choice, and self-determination so often missing from other aspects of their lives.

Having an understanding of the meaning of leisure, play, and recreation can enhance collaboration, planning, and fostering of opportunities for individual choices. With more thought and attention being given to recreation programs and services that provide opportunities for all abilities and interests, people with disabilities will have access to the same benefits of leisure that others have.

Leisure is an important aspect of a high quality of life.

Every artist was first an amateur.
—Ralph Waldo Emerson

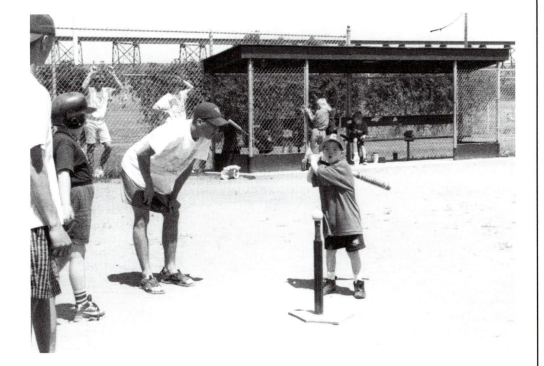

Assignment

You Can't Take Them Away!

Complete this exercise in a small group. Think about some of the most enjoyable experiences or activities in your life. Close your eyes and really visualize what those experiences were or are like. What do they it sound like? smell like? look like? Write these activities on the blanks here. These can be considered important leisure experiences in your life.

_____

_____

_____

_____

Your group members are now going to "take away" your experiences listed above. You have two minutes to convince them why you need those experiences back. What were some of the reasons you gave for the importance of these leisure experiences in your life? Write them here.

_____

_____

_____

_____

Imagine how you would be a different person if you had not had these leisure experiences in your life. Describe how you would be different.

_____

_____

_____

_____

For some people with disabilities, opportunities to have leisure experiences like yours may have been limited. How can *you* change that?

_____

_____

_____

_____

Chapter 2

What Is Inclusion?

Inclusion is defined as "being a member of a larger whole; to encompass or embrace as part of a whole" *(Webster's College Dictionary)*. This definition reflects the philosophy of including people with disabilities into recreation opportunities in our communities. People with disabilities can enrich the recreation experience of others and add healthy diversity to a program. It is important to understand that inclusion means not only *physical* inclusion, but also *social* inclusion. People with disabilities, like all people, want to meet new friends, have opportunities for social interaction, and be a functional participant in a recreation activity. Physical *and* social inclusion must be fostered for these needs to be met.

Inclusion
Process nurtured by professionals, families, and friends in recreation and leisure settings

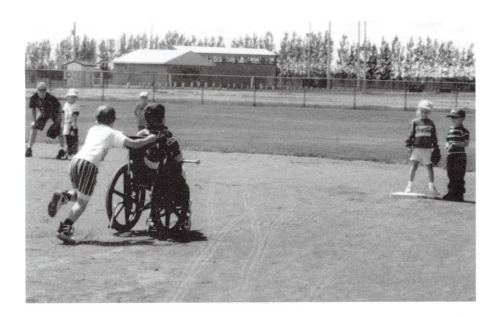

Inclusion Is...

...Having the same choices and opportunities in recreation activities that other people have

Just because a participant may learn slowly or use a wheelchair does not mean he or she should not be able to participate in the same activities as everyone else. An accommodation may be needed to allow for inclusive participation, but the accommodation itself should not deter the opportunity to participate. If a recreation activity is an interest of the participant, then the opportunity needs to exist. The idea of inclusion is to be able to choose what we want to do based on interest.

...Being accepted and appreciated for who you are

People with disabilities have many strengths to add to a recreation program. We often tend to overlook those strengths. People with disabilities will tell you what they can and cannot do.

My daughter with Down syndrome would play at our neighborhood playground when other kids were there, but she was always on the edge, never involved with the kids. Now that she's been included in the neighborhood Girl Scout Troop, the other kids know her and invite her to play on the playground.

Inclusion is being a welcomed participant with friends who share your interests, not your disability.

...Being with friends who share your interests, not your disability

Inclusion is participating in programs where you share the same interests as your friends. The common bond is the recreation activity, not your disability.

...Being a valued customer and a welcomed participant in community recreation programs, regardless of ability level

Inclusion is a choice and an opportunity to open doors to serve more people, regardless of ability level. People with disabilities pay their taxes and dues to the community in which they live. Therefore, they need to be seen as valued members and a welcomed participants.

...Having recreation facilities and areas that are accessible and easy for everyone to use

Inclusion is providing accessible facilities and areas. Accessibility benefits not only people with disabilities, but also older people and parents who use strollers. Accessibility makes everyone's lives easier.

...Providing the necessary individual adaptations, accommodations, and supports so every person can benefit equally from a recreation experience in the community with friends

Inclusion is a process that begins with an individual who may need supports. Providing the individualized supports and accommodations needed by each person is key to successful inclusion.

Things To Avoid When Planning for Inclusion

Inclusion is *not* special, segregated programs.

Avoid putting large groups of people with disabilities in one program

Putting people with disabilities in large groups makes it harder for them to get to know people without disabilities and harder for people without disabilities to get to know them.

Avoid disrupting the natural proportion of individuals with and without disabilities in the community

Programs developed and implemented at your agency should reflect the community. For example, our communities are not only made up of people with disabilities—they are made up of people of all ability levels. Your agency should be offering a variety of programs to meet the needs of your diverse community.

Treat a man as he is, and he will remain as he is. Treat a man as he could be, and he will become what he should be.
—Ralph Waldo Emerson

Avoid special, labeled programs such as "Handicapped Gym Program" or "Bowling for the Mentally Handicapped"

Segregated programs may limit the opportunities for inclusion because the community may view segregated programs as the "choice" for leisure for people with disabilities. Offer an array of choices in recreation activities.

Avoid "caring for" or "looking after" people with disabilities instead of facilitating equal opportunities for equal participation that include risk and challenge

People with disabilities should have the opportunity to take risks and face challenges like everyone else. Challenge is important to a quality leisure experience and people with disabilities have the same right to quality leisure as everyone.

Why Promote Inclusion?

Inclusive recreation opportunities allow people of all ability levels to participate in recreation programs of their choice, based on interest. The process of including people with disabilities into regular recreation programs benefits not only participants *with* disabilities, but also participants *without* disabilities. Many assume that the benefits of inclusion are only experienced by people with disabilities. Inclusive recreation programs prepare people with disabilities for life in an integrated society, and just as importantly, prepare society to accept individual diversity (Dattilo, 2002). Several benefits of inclusive recreation programs follow.

Improved quality of life of all participants

As a result of participation in inclusive leisure opportunities, many people without disabilities report that they experienced personal growth and increased social sensitivity, including improved capacity for compassion, kindness, and respect for others. For people with disabilities, participating in inclusive recreation programs provides opportunities to develop new and to rekindle old friendships, to enhance their self-image by being accepted by others who share their interests, and to develop lifelong functional recreation skills by experiencing challenges of integrated community life (Dattilo, 2002).

Provision of appropriate role models

Inclusive recreation environments provide role models that promote age-appropriate participation patterns for people with disabilities, who may not have much exposure to typical everyday life and its social customs (Dattilo, 2002).

Increased social interaction among participants

In integrated recreation programs, peers without disabilities learn to associate with people different from themselves and usually find that there are more similarities than differences. People with disabilities increase their social skills by interacting with peers without disabilities.

According to Schleien and Green (1992) exposure to integrated recreation services results in a greater understanding and acceptance of individuals with varying backgrounds and ability levels, creating the potential for integration to have a positive impact on the social development of all individuals. Therefore, the focus is on the activity and actions of the activity, rather than on the disability and the actions of the disability.

Benefits of Inclusion
- Improves quality of life
- Provides appropriate role models
- Increases social interaction
- Increases positive attitudes
- Increases independence

How we spend our days is, of course, how we spend our lives.
—Anne Dillard

Increased positive attitudes toward people with disabilities and a better understanding of specific disabilities

According to Schleien (1993) recreation professionals can take an active role in reducing social stigmas associated with persons with disabilities by emphasizing similarities rather than differences. Through ongoing sensitivity training, education, and structured interaction, attitudes toward people with disabilities can become more positive. Your staff need to be given the appropriate training and support to learn more about people with disabilities and to feel comfortable when interacting with them.

Increased independence among participants

In inclusive community recreation programs, participants with disabilities strive to be as independent as possible. They want to be seen as individuals with opportunities to make their own choices. The more people with disabilities are involved in inclusive environments, the better the opportunity for them to develop independent skills.

Inclusion is a process that starts with each individual. Inclusion works by determining how best that person can be fully included—what skills that person needs, what input the staff and participants require, what supports are necessary, and how that support generalizes to other environments (Berger, 1994).

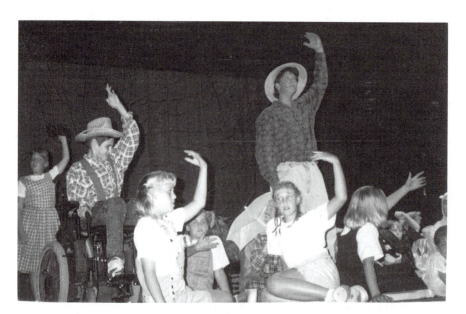

It's the Person First—Then the Disability

If you saw a person in a wheelchair unable to get up the stairs into a building, would you say, "There is a handicapped person unable to find a ramp?" Or would you say, "There is a person with a disability handicapped by an inaccessible building?"

What is the proper way to speak to or about someone who does not have a disability?

Consider how you would introduce someone—Jane Doe—who doesn't have a disability. You would give her name, where she lives, what she does or what she is interested in—she likes swimming, or eating Mexican food, or watching Brad Pitt movies.

The worst sin toward our fellow creatures is not to hate them, but to be indifferent to them; that's the essence of inhumanity.
—George Bernard Shaw

What do you see first?
   The wheelchair?
   The physical problem?
   The person?

Why say it differently for a person with a disability?

Every person is made up of many characteristics—mental as well as physical—and few want to be identified only by their ability to play tennis or by their love for fried onions or by the mole on their face. Those are just parts of us.

In speaking or writing, remember that children or adults with disabilities are like everyone else—except they happen to have a disability. Focusing on the person, not the disability, is one of the keys to successful inclusion; however, additional information on types of disabilities can be found in Appendix B.

Label jars, not people.
—Unknown

Tips for Improving Language Related to Disabilities and Handicaps

- Speak of the person first, then the disability.
- Emphasize abilities, not limitations.
- Do not label people as part of a disability group—don't say "the disabled." Say "people with disabilities."
- Don't give excessive praise or attention to a person with a disability and don't patronize.
- Choice and independence are important; let the person do or speak for himself or herself as much as possible.
- If addressing an adult say "Bill" instead of "Billy."
- A *disability* is a functional limitation that interferes with a person's ability to walk, hear, learn, etc. A *handicap* describes a situation or barrier imposed by society, the environment, or oneself.
- Focus on what the person can do and not on what they can't do. Each participant can add excitement and variety to the group and/or program.

Instead of...	Say...
disabled or handicapped child	child with a disability
palsied, spastic	person with cerebral palsy
afflicted, suffers from	person who has
mute or dumb	without speech, nonverbal
slow	developmental delay
crazy, insane	mental illness
confined to a wheelchair	uses a wheelchair
retarded, mental	person with retardation
mongoloid	with Down syndrome
normal	without a disability
crippled	has a physical disability
invalid	paralyzed
the blind	visually impaired

A *disability* is a functional limitation that interferes with abilities.

A *handicap* is a barrier imposed by society.

Assignment

Language and Behavior Awareness Survey

This survey is an excellent tool to use when training staff on inclusion and how to communicate and interact with people with disabilities. The answers begin on page 14.

1. From the following items, check the item that you believe describes where the word "handicapped" comes from:

    _____A. Golf, where poorer players are given an advantage to allow them to compete

    _____B. Horse racing, where faster horses must carry heavy weights

    _____C. Beggars, who held caps in their hands

    _____D. None of the above

2. Place a check by the terms that you recognize.

    _____A. Blind as a bat

    _____B. Not playing with a full deck

    _____C. The blind leading the blind

    _____D. A cripple (in baseball or other sports)

    _____E. Stone deaf

3. When speaking to a person who has a disability, it is rude to use words that reference their impairment. For example, asking a person who is blind if they "see" your point or asking a person in a wheelchair if they would like to go for a "walk."

    True_____   False_____

4. When listening to a person whose speech is difficult to understand, the average person will

    _____A. Say he or she does not understand.

    _____B. Pretend to understand.

    _____C. Make an excuse to end the conversation.

5. It is impolite during a conversation with someone who is blind to look directly into his or her eyes as you would someone who is not blind.

    True_____   False_____

6. What should you do when a person with a hearing impairment asks to have a statement repeated?

    _____A. Repeat the statement.

    _____B. Repeat the statement more slowly and in a louder voice.

    _____C. Rephrase the statement.

7. When holding a face-to-face conversation with someone using a wheelchair, what should you do?

    _____A. Find a chair and sit down so you are both on the same level.

    _____B. Step back so he or she can see you more comfortably.

    _____C. Avoid leaning on or touching the wheelchair.

    _____D. All of the above

8. The only kind of dogs legally allowed into hotels and restaurants to assist persons with disabilities are dog guides for people who have vision impairments.

   True_____   False_____

9. If someone is using a sign language interpreter, it is proper to address questions and responses to the interpreter so he or she can relay them to the person who is deaf.

   True_____   False_____

10. When meeting a person who is blind, it is proper etiquette to announce who you are even if the person has met you before.

   True_____   False_____

11. When meeting a person who has an artificial right hand, it would be proper etiquette to
   _____A. Reach out with your right hand to shake theirs as if there was no difference.
   _____B. Reach out with your left hand.
   _____C. Pause, waiting for the person to initiate contact.

12. When you are unsure of what to do in a situation with someone with a disability, it is permissible to admit you are unsure and ask the person for advice.

   True_____   False_____

13. The discomfort one feels in the presence of someone with a disability never really goes away.

   True_____   False_____

14. Under what circumstances would it be permissible to interact with a guide dog of a person who is visually impaired or blind?

Adapted from a survey written by Richard Pimentel, Senior Partner, Milt Wright & Associates, Inc. Organizational Design, Training and Development. 800-626-3939, www.miltwright.com

Source: The Americans With Disabilities Act: Making the ADA Work For You Trainer's Manual, *Copyright 1992, Milt Wright & Associates, Inc.*

Answers to Language and Behavior Awareness Survey

1. C

   Old English concept of when beggars held caps in their hands on the streets, begging for money. The term "cap in hand" became "handicapped."

2. We are sure you could think of others. Negative stereotypes of people with disabilities live on in our everyday language.

3. False

   Talk to the person with a disability as you would someone without a disability. The disability is just a part of the person.

4. B

   Most people will pretend to understand for fear of not knowing what to do or embarrassing the person with a speech impairment.

5. False

   Again, talk to the person with a disability just like you would talk to others. If you look other people in the eyes or focus on their nose, then do the same for the person who is blind. There is no special way to talk to people who are blind or have any other type of disability.

6. A

   It is best to repeat the statement. A louder voice may be more of a squeaking noise, and slowing down is more difficult as the person with a hearing impairment may be reading your lips, and this makes it more difficult to follow your lip movements.

7. D

   Try to be at eye level for the person in a wheelchair. Using these three techniques will make it much easier for the person to focus on you and not strain her or his neck. Also, the wheelchair is an extension of the person and a part of who they are, so do not lean on or touch the chair.

8. False

   Dog guides also assist people who use wheelchairs and people with other disabilities.

9. False

   Always address the person with a hearing impairment. The interpreter will interpret everything you are saying, so make sure your conversation is with the person with the hearing impairment. The interpreter is your communication link to the person with a hearing impairment. If you need to talk with the interpreter, you can do so before or after the program. Let the interpreter know you need to speak to him or her alone.

10. True

    Eventually, they will get to know you by the sound of your voice. Most people meet others twice before they remember names, and the person who is blind is no exception.

11. A

    Extend whatever hand you shake with and the person with the artificial hand will extend the hand she or he wishes to shake with, or may just nod her or his head in greeting.

12. True

    Always ask. People with disabilities would rather have you ask them than assume or pretend. Asking will only make the conversation and the time together less intimidating.

13. Only you know what your comfort level is and will be around people with disabilities. We hope the discomfort will go away, and it does for most people.

14. Out of harness, but still ask permission. Even though the dog is out of harness, it is still polite to ask.

Chapter 3

What Is Physical Accessibility and How Is It Accomplished?

What Is Physical Accessibility?

Physical accessibility means recreation facilities and areas are barrier-free and people with disabilities can approach, enter, and use them unimpeded. The following diagram illustrates the framework in which accessibility can be accomplished.

> Approach ⟶ Enter ⟶ Use ⟶ Conveniences

Approach

People with disabilities should be able to approach a recreation facility without encountering obstacles. For example, providing curb cuts near the facility or ramps will allow for accessible routes of travel. Accessible, clearly marked, and well-designed parking spaces are necessary as well.

Enter

Once a person with a disability approaches a recreation facility, the entrance must be accessible as well. Accessible entrances must be clearly marked. Doors that pull open easily or a bell that rings for access are examples of accessible entrances. Doors must be wide and light enough and thresholds low enough to allow entrance. Double doors must not impede entrance.

Use

Once inside a recreation area or facility, people with disabilities must be able to use the facility. Are the restrooms accessible? Can a person with a disability access the concession area? Is playground equipment accessible? If a person can approach and enter a recreation area, but not use it like their peers, then it is not accessible. Often to use a facility or program effectively some accommodations or supports may be needed. Examples of accommodations include an interpreter, assistance from a volunteer, or a piece of adaptive equipment. Accommodations and supports will be discussed in detail in Chapter 4.

Conveniences

Many accommodations available today would be wonderful to have, and agencies could provide many additional services. But the bottom line must be: Can a person

Things do not change, we do.
—Henry David Thoreau

When planning for physical accessibility, ask the following questions:
- Can the person *approach* the facility?
- Can the person *enter* the facility?
- Can the person *use* the facility once inside?
- What *conveniences* would facilitate inclusion?

Examples of universal accessibility design concepts when planning a new playground

- Surfacing under playground components allows for use of wheelchairs or strollers.
- Ramps and transfer systems allow access to varying heights of equipment.
- Overhead play components (e.g., monkey bars) at varying heights to accommodate all sizes and abilities.
- A variety of swing sets are provided in the same swing bay area,
- Play components that use varied skills (e.g., social, physical, cognitive) are designed into the playground.

with a disability *approach*, *enter*, and *use* this facility and program? If so, accommodations provided beyond that can be considered conveniences. For example, an agency could install an automatic door opener, but because an accessible entrance could be created by having a door that is lightweight to open and a lever handle that is easy to grasp, this would be considered a convenience.

In summary, the level at which facilities need to be accessible should be based on the belief that inclusion is socially and economically feasible and desirable. Playgrounds, parks, gymnasiums, trails, pathways, and other recreation facilities should be barrier-free for everyone, regardless of ability level. Facilities and areas need to be *universally accessible*.

What Is Universal Accessibility?

Universal accessibility is a design approach that ensures maximum inclusion and participation by everyone. It is based on the belief that people who have disabilities should have the same access to buildings and facilities that other citizens enjoy. People who believe this promote universally accessible designs for all new apartments, town houses, public buildings, washrooms, workplaces, and parks and recreation facilities. They include accessibility in all remodeling and renovation projects.

Physical accessibility has become a common concern among recreation professionals since the passage of the Americans With Disabilities Act (ADA). This legislation has caused an increased awareness of the need to serve all community members in parks and recreation facilities *and* programs, including people with disabilities.

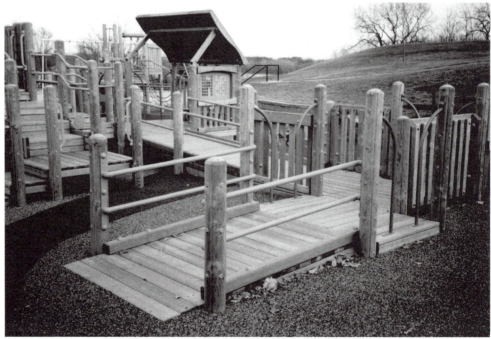

Photo courtesy of Eden Prairie, MN Parks, Recreation, and Natural Resources Department

With an accessible playground in our neighborhood, I can now play with my child like other parents can.
—Parent who uses a wheelchair

What Is the Americans With Disabilities Act?

The Americans with Disabilities Act (P.L. 101-336) was passed in 1990. The purpose of the ADA is to end discrimination against individuals with disabilities and to welcome them into all walks of life so they may enjoy the same privileges as other citizens. Although many people tend to think of ADA as focusing on physical accessibility, it also mandates program accessibility. The ADA applies to

- Public-funded services (local, county, district, state, federal)

- Not-for-profit agencies or services (e.g., YMCA, Girl Scouts, camps, Easter Seals)

- Private for-profit enterprises (e.g., bowling alleys, movie theaters, amusements parks)

The ADA covers anyone who has a disability, has a record of a disability, or is regarded as having a disability, and anyone who may face discrimination due to their relationship with persons with disabilities.

No qualified individual with a disability shall, on the basis of disability, be excluded from participation in or be denied the benefits of the services, programs, or activities of public entity, or be subjected to discrimination by any public entity. (28 CFR 35.130)

Although the ADA requirements vary according to type (e.g., state, private) and size of the agency, many guidelines outlined by ADA would be beneficial for any recreation agency to follow.

Individual rights are not subject to a public vote; a majority has no right to vote away the rights of a minority; the political function of rights is precisely to protect minorities from oppression by majorities (and the smallest minority on earth is the individual).
—Ayn Rand

Five Major Titles of the ADA

Title I: Employment
Employers may not discriminate against individuals with disabilities in the workplace. This includes all employment actions.

Title IIa: State/Local Government
Public entities/local government shall not exclude an individual with a disability from participation in, or the benefits of, programs, services, and activities.

Title IIb: Transportation
Governments that provide transportation must assure that all services are readily accessible to and usable by individuals with disabilities.

Title III: Businesses/Public Accommodations
Businesses that provide goods, services, or facilities to the public must not discriminate on the basis of disability in the provision of their services.

Title IV: Communications
Public and private entities must make all services accessible to persons with communication impairments.

Title V: Miscellaneous
This title covers a variety of issues, including regulations and enforcement.

What Are the Standards for Physical Accessibility?

The Architectural Barriers Act (ABA) of 1968 (P.L. 90-480) was the first federal law requiring facility access for people with physical disabilities, stating that "any building or facility constructed in whole or in part by federal funds must be made accessible and usable by the physically handicapped." The Architectural and Transportation Barriers Compliance Board (Access Board), created by this legislation, issued minimum guidelines to ensure that buildings, facilities, rail passenger cars, and vehicles were accessible and usable by people with disabilities.

Following is a list of standards that will assist in improving facility design to meet the needs of all people. The set of standards you use depends on your agency and your funding. Whichever you use, you must stay consistent. If state and federal standards differ, *always comply with the more stringent standards*. The Access Board is

Whenever you must decide which set of standards to use in making your agency accessible, always choose the most stringent standards.

currently developing a combined set of standards. Check the Access Board website for the current status of the combined standards (http://www.access-board.gov).

The American National Standards Institute

If we did all the things we are capable of, we would literally astound ourselves.
—Thomas Edison

First developed in 1961, the American National Standards Institute (ANSI) 117.1 was the first building standard to address issues of accessibility. The standards presented in 117.1 were developed through consensus by a committee of over 50 organizations representing associations of individuals with disabilities, rehabilitation professionals, designers, builders, manufacturers, and government agencies. Two thirds of states currently incorporate or reference the 117.1 standard or other documents, such as the model building codes of the Uniform Federal Accessibility Standards (UFAS), in their building codes (Goltsman, Gilbert & Wohlford, 1993).

Uniform Federal Accessibility Standards

The Uniform Federal Accessibility Standards (UFAS) define the standards for design, construction, and alteration of buildings to meet the requirements of the Architectural Barriers Act (ABA) Access Guidelines. UFAS references the ANSI 117.1 standard and is based on the Minimum Guidelines and Requirements for Accessible Design (MGRAD), developed by the Architectural and Transportation Barriers Compliance Board to provide direction to federal agencies that oversee federally owned, leased, or financed buildings. UFAS is the title of the standards actually adopted by those agencies. Recreational and civic buildings and sites that require public access or that might serve as a place of employment for people with disabilities, are among the facilities addressed in these standards (Goltsman, Gilbert & Wohlford, 1993).

The ADA Accessibility Guidelines (ADAAG) cover facilities in the private sector (e.g., public accommodations, commercial facilities) and public sector (e.g., state and local government facilities).

The accessibility guidelines under ABA cover facilities in the federal sector or facilities funded by the federal government.

A new federal ruling (pending March, 2003) will combine the two laws under one common set of criteria for accessibility.

Americans With Disabilities Act Accessibility Guidelines

The most current and the most preferred standards to use are the Americans With Disabilities Act Accessibility Guidelines (ADAAG). In regard to physical accessibility, ADA extends the intent of the Architectural Barriers Act to cover all public facilities regardless of federal funding, including restaurants, hospitals, movie theaters, medical and law offices, and retail stores. The sections of the Act that address these issues are Title II (Public Services and Public Transportation) and Title III (Public Accommodations and Services; Goltsman, Gilbert & Wohlford, 1993). In addition, ADAAG includes guidelines for outdoor recreation areas and facilities. These guidelines, some of which are still being developed, address areas such as trails, fishing piers, swimming pools, and gymnasiums.

The ADAAG and UFAS survey tools and guidelines are excellent resources to use when evaluating your agency for accessibility. Whichever survey is used, it is important that you adhere to the same guidelines for each facility.

How Do I Know If Our Facilities and Programs Are Accessible?

The ADA mandates planning for accessibility in facilities and programs, and many parks and recreation agencies have already taken steps toward this. When planning and preparing to welcome all people, and to comply with ADA, the following principles will assist you in the process.

- Designate an ADA/Accessibility Coordinator whose roles include over-seeing the planning, training, implementation, and evaluation of making your agency welcoming and providing a single point of contact to the public.

- Provide public notice. Let interested people know who the ADA/Accessibility Coordinator is and make sure the public is aware of anticipated compliance steps.

- Contact and involve interested people who have disabilities, as well as advocates who work with people with disabilities.

- Conduct a comprehensive *self-evaluation*, noting where your agency is already accessible and where future changes are needed to achieve physical and programmatic accessibility.

- Prepare an *accessibility plan* that describes necessary changes, how they will be corrected, a time frame for completion, and the responsible party. (***Note***: ADA mandates a transition plan. However, given that the law was passed over a decade ago, the authors feel that agencies should be well past the transition plan phase, and instead have an active and ongoing access plan in place.)

- Develop a grievance procedure for handling complaints.

- Conduct sensitivity training for *all* employees.

- Review employment provisions of ADA to ensure compliance.

- Ensure that individuals with disabilities can readily communicate with your agency (e.g., TDD/TTY, relay service, e-mail, website).

- Be sure that all new facilities and major alterations meet ADAAG or UFAS standards for accessibility.

- Review programs and services to assure they are being provided in the most integrated setting possible.

- Use representatives from disability organizations whenever possible to advise your department/agency on how to provide program access in the most integrated setting possible.

- Keep communication open with all representatives assisting you with this process. Listen to all concerns and issues presented to you.

Completing an accessibility survey in a wheelchair is very enlightening for most people. Barriers that seem insignificant, such as a raised threshold, can actually bar access.

How Do I Complete a Self-Evaluation and an Accessibility Plan?

This section will assist you in completing a self-evaluation and developing a plan for accessibility. The information provided enables both public and private agencies to evaluate their current programs, activities, services, benefits, goods, and privileges to identify potential structural and nonstructural barriers that prevent equal participation and enjoyment for persons with disabilities.

The Self-Evaluation Process

The self-evaluation process will help you to identify barriers that impede inclusion of people with disabilities (e.g., communication, registration, physical access, transportation). The access plan will identify the necessary steps to achieve physical accessibility of all facilities. Follow these steps to complete a self-evaluation.

☐ List all programs, services, and activities you provide (inventory).

☐ Concisely describe each program, service, or activity.

☐ Collect and document the policies, procedures, and priorities that govern your day-to-day operation (written and unwritten).

☐ Analyze how current policies, procedures, and practices (or lack thereof) affect or impact individuals with disabilities.

☐ Determine if any barriers are physical and can be solved through nonstructural changes.

☐ Identify solutions to modify existing policies, procedures, and practices to allow for full inclusion of people with disabilities.

☐ Consult with interested persons, especially people with disabilities, on identified barriers and solutions, as well as other self-evaluation data.

☐ Keep a copy of your self-evaluation on file.

The Plan for Accessibility

The access plan is a process to identify the necessary steps to achieve physical accessibility of all facilities. Follow the eight steps outlined on the next page to complete a plan for accessibility.

Suggestions for Improving Access for People With Disabilities

Although the self-evaluation and accessibility plan identify specific structural changes an agency must make, the following suggestions are helpful when planning and implementing physical accessibility. (***Note***: These suggestions do not guarantee compliance with ADA—it is the agency's responsibility to understand the specific requirements of ADA.)

Improving Accessibility for Mobility Impairments

Path of Travel

When planning for accessibility for people with mobility impairments, pay attention to the following:
• Path of travel
• Doors
• Stairs, ramps, elevators
• Restrooms

• A pathway should connect separate buildings or activity areas within the same site.

• Designate parking for people with disabilities as close as possible to the accessible entrance.

• A smooth, firm pathway of nonslip material at least 36 inches wide, with no unramped changes of level should lead from the parking area to the entrance.

Steps for Completing a Plan for Accessiblitiy

Step One
Identify the facilities owned or leased by your agency.

Step Two
Survey the facilities identified. Record measurements of building elements that are key to achieving access.

Step Three
Compare the building survey results with the appropriate standards for accessibility.

Step Four
Determine if any structural barriers exist. Ask people with disabilities to help make this judgment.

Step Five
Develop solutions to overcome the barriers identified.

Step Six
Develop an access plan. This plan should include the following:

- The structural barrier, what will be done to overcome the barrier, and the standard that will be met (ADAAG or UFAS)

- Estimated cost of the solution

- Reason why proposed the solution was chosen

- Priorities for implementation

- Timetable for implementation

- Name of person responsible for implementation

Step Seven
Identify the structural barriers and solutions not proposed to be implemented because of a determination of "undue burden" (state and local government) or because a solution is not "readily achievable" (private businesses). Undue burden will be tested by the courts, but the conditions necessary to prove undue burden are difficult to meet. The elements of the test for undue burden include

- Undue economic burden

- Undue administrative burden

- Fundamental alteration in the nature of the program, service, or activity of the facility

In general, the whole scope and nature of the services you offer should be analyzed on a case-by-case basis to determine if accommodations are indeed undue burden. Publicly funded agencies (e.g., those services that are paid for by tax dollars and that have the purpose of serving all people) are required to make every effort to adhere to the ADA, except in rare cases.

Step Eight
Retain a copy of the accessibility plan on file and monitor its implementation.

The plan for accessibility describes the necessary changes needed by an agency, how the changes will be made, the time frame for completion, and the responsible party.

The reward of a thing well done is having done it.
—Ralph Waldo Emerson

A wheelchair requires a 5-foot diameter space to make a 360-degree turn.

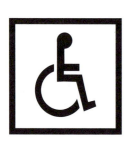

- A 36-inch wide path of travel with no unramped changes of level should connect activity areas within the building.

- Securely anchor carpets and mats to floor surfaces.

- Rearrange furniture and remove obstacles for a 36-inch clear path of travel, and a 5-foot diameter space wherever a 360-degree turn is necessary for wheelchair users.

- Replace widely spaced grates with ones with less than one half inch wide openings.

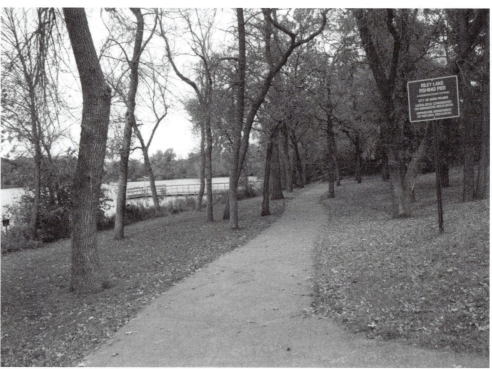

Photo courtesy of Eden Prairie, MN Parks, Recreation, and Natural Resources Department

Doors

- At inaccessible entrances, place signs bearing the International Symbol of Accessibility and an arrow indicating the location of the accessible entrance.

- Doorways should have 32 inches minimum clearance.

- Replace doorknobs with lever or loop handles.

- Remove or lower thresholds, or add a wedge on both sides of threshold to ease movement and prevent tripping.

- Install doormats one half inch thick or less.

Stairs, Ramps, and Elevators

- Hold meetings/events in spaces that do not require stairs.

- Add nonslip treads to stairs.

- Ramps should be sloped at 1:12 or less.

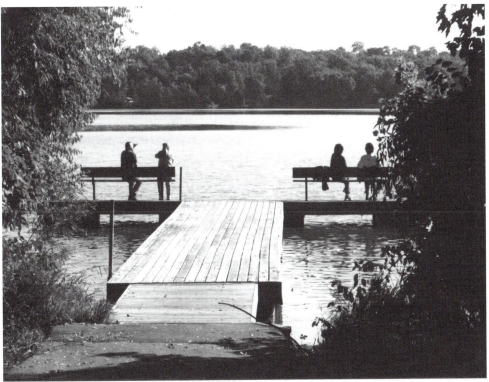

Photo courtesy of Eden Prairie, MN Parks, Recreation, and Natural Resources Department

Restrooms

- Install a handle on the inside of the stall door.

- Replace stall door hinges with the self-closing type.

- Relocate paper towel and other dispensers to a maximum of 42 inches above the floor.

- Provide knee space below the sink at 27 inches high, 30 inches wide, and 22 inches deep.

- Enlarge the stall to accommodate grab bars and an accessible toilet.

- Provide a 5-foot turning space in the communal part of the restroom.

- Install paddle faucet controls.

- Insulate the pipes under the sink.

Note: Renovations (such as installing lifts or elevators, renovating toilet facilities, or building a long ramp) will require expert consultation and a contractor. Monitor the design and construction. Involve people with disabilities in planning the renovations.

Improving Accessibility for Hearing/Speech Impairments

Telephone Amplifiers

The telephone company can install amplification devices on pay phones. For amplification on your phones contact your local phone company.

Man who says it cannot be done should not interrupt man who is doing it.
—Chinese proverb

If you cannot hear well or you cannot speak clearly, improving accessibility means improving ways to communicate.

An *Assistive Listening System* (ALS) is designed to help people with hearing loss to improve auditory access in large areas. It augments a public address system.

Assistive Listening Systems

If your agency has a meeting room, theater, or auditorium, an assistive listening system will enhance the sound for people who are hard of hearing.

Real-Time Reporters

Real-time reporters type what is said in a meeting, and the text is displayed on video monitor or projection screen.

Telecommunication Display Device (TDD) or Teletypewriter (TTY)

A TDD or TTY is a portable electronic machine used with a telephone. The TDD/TTY has a visual display and/or printer so that both the caller and the receiver can type and read their conversation. When you install a TDD/TTY, be sure to train your employees on its use and to publicize its availability.

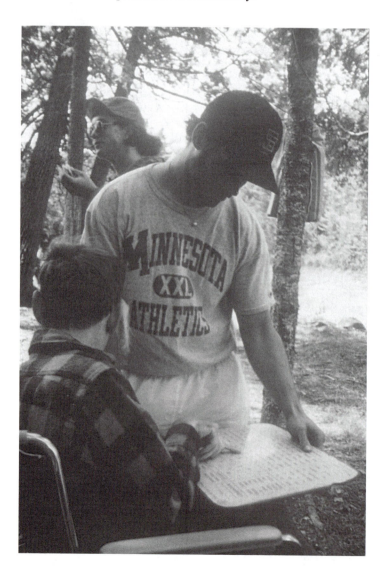

Telecommunication Relay Services

Telecommunication relay services enable someone using a TDD/TTY to communicate with someone using a telephone. Using a TDD/TTY, voice operators at the relay service act as a communication bridge between hearing people and people who are deaf or hard of hearing. Every state has a mandated relay service system that is easily accessible. Contact http://www.neca.org for complete information. (NECA is the National Exchange Carrier Association. It plays an important role in administration of the telecommunication relay system.)

Interpreters

People who are deaf or hard of hearing often request interpreters to participate in conversations, meetings, activities, and events. Sign language interpreters can use American Sign Language (ASL) or Signed English. Oral interpreters paraphrase or mouth silently the spoken message and voice-interpret the speech of a person who is deaf or hard of hearing. The person who is deaf or hard of hearing should be consulted as to the type of interpreting they need.

American Sign Language is the 4th most commonly used language in the United States.
—National Institute on Deafness and Other Communication Disorders

Interpreters can work comfortably for about 45 minutes at a stretch. To provide quality services, two interpreters are generally needed for assignments lasting over two hours with at least one 10 to 15 minute break each.

Emergency Warning Systems

People who are deaf and hard of hearing may need alarms they can see. Emergency alarms, therefore, must be both audible and visual. Audible and visual signals should operate simultaneously (e.g., a lighted exit sign that flashes and beeps when the alarm system is activated).

Vision alarms are effective only when they are within the vision range of people who are deaf or hard of hearing. Flashing white lights are the most effective way to catch the attention of someone with a hearing impairment.

Improving Accessibility for Visual Impairments

People who are blind or visually impaired confront many hazards in the environment. To detect obstacles in the path of travel, some people sweep a long cane from side to side along the ground. Following are some ways to create a more accessible environment for people with visual disabilities.

People with visual impairments have a wide range of abilities, from partially sighted to total blindness, from lack of depth perception to lack of peripheral vision.

- Remove protruding objects, such as wall-mounted telephones and drinking fountains, or recess them into the wall to widen the passageway.

- Place handrails on both sides of stairs and ramps. Add a 1-inch strip of contrasting color to the nosing of each step to help people with limited sight or depth perception see the stair edge.

- Avoid reorganizing storage areas or furniture frequently.

- Improve lighting within the facility, especially in stairwells.

- Use high contrast colors in decorating the facility.

- Floors, sidewalks, stairs, and ramps should be covered or constructed with a nonslip material.

10% of students with significant vision impairments use Braille; 25% use large print.
—Lighthouse International

As more people use the Web to learn about recreation opportunities, it is critical that your agency website is accessible to people with vision impairments.

- Secure the edges of carpets and mats to the floor.

- Install edge strips where floor surfaces change.

- Install tactile floor numbers in raised print and Braille on both sides of elevator door jams and on the control panel.

- Avoid installation of solid glass doors. If they are already installed, place a color decal on windows adjacent to glass doors to distinguish between the two.

- Install signs that have large print, raised lettering, and Braille. Light letters on dark background are easiest to see. Tactile and low vision signage should be placed on the wall next to the door opening, not on the door itself.

- Install audible signals in elevators to indicate the opening and closing of the doors and the passage of floors.

The following provisions can assist in making information about your agency's programs, services, location, proximity to public transportation, and hours of operation accessible to people who are blind or visually impaired.

- Provide large-print materials, double-spaced and printed on a high-contrast background.

- Provide materials in Braille if possible.

- Provide information on audiotapes, computer disks, or on a website. Some people who are blind or visually impaired cannot or prefer not to read Braille or large print and find tapes more useful. Many people with vision impairments have computers that can enlarge written material provided to them on disk or on a webpage.

- If materials for people who are blind or visually impaired are not available, designate someone to be a reader.

What you do speaks so loudly that I cannot hear what you say.
—Ralph Waldo Emerson

Physical accessibility—making facilities barrier-free—is just one part of facilitating inclusion.

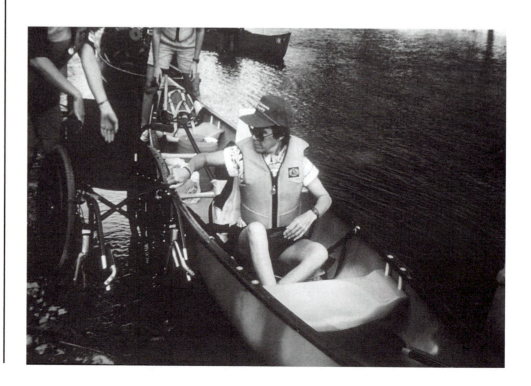

Accessibility: Points to Remember

- Get input from people with disabilities.

- Planning is critical. Develop a team of personnel knowledgeable about the subject, including people with disabilities.

- Consider all types of disabilities—vision, hearing, mobility, coordination, cognitive—when planning for accessibility.

- New structures have to be fully, not partially, accessible.

- Keep in mind whether the participants using your services are adults or children. The standards are based on adults and you have to adapt them for children. Access standards that consider the size of children are available on the U.S. Access Board website (http://www.access-board.gov).

- A new structure is likely to have a useful life of at least 40 years. Consider the potential users in its lifetime.

- Consider accessibility as a regular part of the maintenance and improvement of a facility and check the federal and state codes when undertaking such work.

- Keep in mind that with respect to older buildings program accessibility puts the emphasis on the program or services, not the structure.

- Check with your state law on access. If you have state standards, you must use whichever standards are more stringent between the state and federal.

- Think functionally in terms of people approaching, entering, and using a structure independently, safely, and conveniently.

- Utilize solutions that, while solving the problem for one group of persons with disabilities, do not create a problem for another. For example, curb ramps should have a different texture from sidewalk so that persons who are visually impaired can detect the change of surface and realize they are in the street.

- Be creative. Some of the best solutions to physical accessibility problems are free or very inexpensive. Involve people with disabilities, staff who regularly use the facility, and other program participants to brainstorm possible accommodations.

It's not that I'm smart, it's just that I stay with problems longer.
—Albert Einstein

Improving accessibility varies depending on the type of impairment—physical, hearing, speech, or vision. Other accommodations may be needed for people with cognitive or intellectual impairments as well.

Assignment

Complete a Physical Accessibility Survey

Go to the webpage of the U.S. Access Board (http://www.access-board.gov). Under the "Publications" link you will find a list of guidelines and survey forms that you will need to conduct a thorough accessibility evaluation of a building or outdoor facility. The forms were developed based on the requirements of the Americans with Disabilities Act (ADAAG) and the Uniform Federal Accessibility Standards (UFAS).

Determine which set of standards to use, based on your agency and funding source. Remember, ADAAG standards are the most current and comprehensive. Be sure to review any existing accessibility plans your agency may have completed. Also, determine the ADA/Access Coordinator in your agency.

It is likely that you will need to reproduce the survey forms several times to completely evaluate a single building or outdoor facility. Once you have obtained the necessary survey forms, you will need to assess one of the recreation facilities owned or used by your agency. It is very helpful to use a wheelchair during your assessment. Many overlooked barriers in the facility will become evident as you travel through it in a wheelchair. Compare the results of your assessment with the ADAAG or UFAS standards.

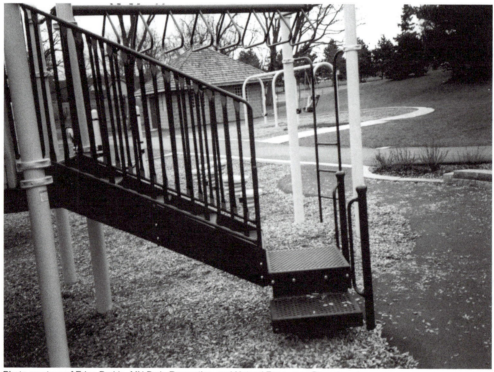

Photo courtesy of Eden Prairie, MN Park, Recreation, and Natural Resources Department

Chapter 4

What Is Program Accessibility and How Is It Accomplished?

What Is Program Accessibility?

Program accessibility is designing recreation programs and activities so people with disabilities can actively and socially participate in them. It involves providing necessary supports and services so people with disabilities can pursue the activities of their choice.

According to Schleien (1993), although recent laws mandate agencies to accommodate individuals of varying abilities, both architecturally and programmatically, often these agencies have only removed architectural barriers. Without program access, participants without disabilities continue to view their peers with disabilities and integration efforts negatively (Schleien, 1993).

Chapter 3 briefly illustrated a process by which accessibility should be accomplished. Whereas the *approach* and *enter* steps relate primarily to physical accessibility, the next two steps, *use* and *conveniences*, relate more to program and service accessibility. Once people with disabilities have approached and entered the facility, the next step is providing the necessary and appropriate accommodations to allow for usage of the facility (e.g., large-print brochures, interpreters, one-on-one assistance, relocation of a program), and more importantly, social inclusion in the activity.

Program accessibility means providing supports and accommodations so people with disabilities can pursue their leisure choices, beyond making the space physically accessible.

Approach $\longrightarrow$ Enter $\longrightarrow$ Use $\longrightarrow$ Conveniences

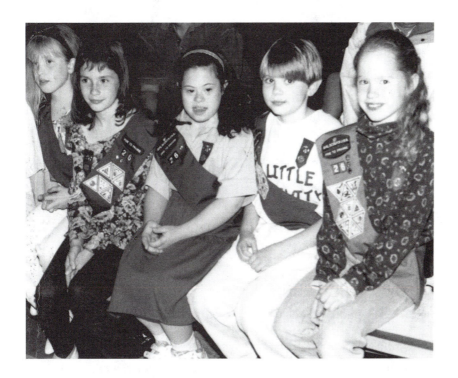

Because we live in a world of change and diversity, we are privileged to enter into a diversity of visions, and beyond that, to include them in the range of responsible caring.
—Mary Catherine Bateson

The Inclusion Process

For inclusion efforts to be successful, a process must be followed to identify and to address the needs of people with disabilities. Having a clear process for planning will provide the structure and support needed to ensure full participation (Hutchison & McGill, 1992).

A variety of strategies within the process can be used to facilitate and to encourage the inclusion of people with disabilities, as well as to create accessible programs, services, and welcoming facilities. The following is a step-by-step process for inclusion that can be adapted to meet the particular needs within an agency. This process assumes that your agency has established programs in which inclusion can occur.

Step One: Program Promotion

When promoting programs through brochures, flyers, and newsletters, all program materials should include nondiscriminatory and/or welcoming statements that communicate to participants what kind of support is available to assist them and how to request supports or accommodations that may be needed. This statement addresses the willingness of the agency to work with everyone, regardless of ability level.

(Agency name) is committed to providing reasonable accommodations and accessibility for all residents. If you have any specific needs for participation, please contact (staff person) at (phone number). To ensure that we meet your accessibility needs, a prior contact of (time frame) is desired.

In addition, program promotions should be available in alternate format, such as computer disk, audiotape, or large print. A statement about the availability of alternate formats should be included at the front of the printed material. The publication could also include an easily recognized accessibility symbol.

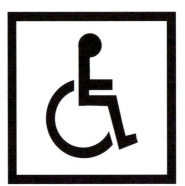

International Symbol of Access

All program promotions should be sent to the general community. Make sure to include

- Individuals with disabilities

- Families of individuals with disabilities

- Schools (regular and special education)

- Advocacy agencies (Arc, independent living centers)

- Human/social service centers, group homes, senior centers

How wonderful it is that nobody need wait a single moment before starting to improve the world.
—Anne Frank

Welcoming statements in agency promotional materials advertise your willingness to provide services to *all* citizens in your community.

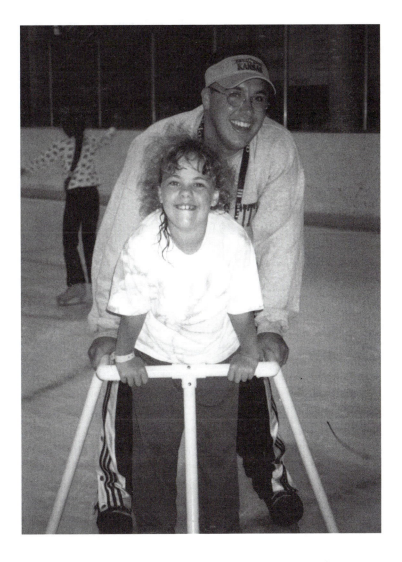

It ain't what you don't know that gets you into trouble, it's what you know for sure that just ain't so.
—Mark Twain

Step Two: Registration Process and Assessment of Needs

People with disabilities register for programs using the same registration process other participants use. Be sure registration locations are physically accessible to all individuals. Identify a staff person to be responsible for inclusion requests. To assist you in effectively meeting the needs of each participant, your agency's registration form should have a statement that identifies the specific needs of a particular participant. For example:

> *Does the participant require any accommodations or have any needs of which we should be aware?*

If this statement is checked "yes," then further information is needed. Either by phone or in person contact the participant or parent/guardian and discuss any accommodations that may be needed. Appendix D has examples of intake forms and specific agency assessment forms to use in identifying needs and accommodations. If talking on the phone is difficult, ask the participant and/or the participant's parent or guardian to meet you at your agency, the program site, or the participant's home to discuss further needs and to arrange a tour of the facilities.

Never assume a person's needs based on disability—always ask. Everyone has unique needs, regardless of disability or ability.

Step Three: Accommodations and Supports

From the information you gathered with the participant intake process, you must determine if any supports or accommodations are needed for the person with a disability

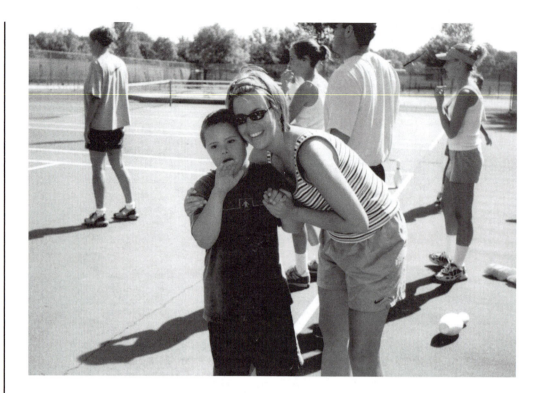

The world is but a canvas to our imagination.
—Henry David Thoreau

to fully participate in the program. Supports and accommodations are merely solutions to meet the needs of an individual participant in the program. There are unlimited numbers of accommodations—the needs of the person with the disability and your creativity are the only limiting factors. Ask the participant first what types of accommodations are needed. The following is a list of some examples of accommodations. Depending on the individual needs of the participant, one or several accommodations may be used.

Accommodations: Equipment and Activity Adaptations

The following is a list of activity or equipment adaptations that could be used when including people with disabilities (Rynders and Schleien, 1991; Schleien, Ray & Green, 1997).

Equipment/materials. Some people with disabilities may need specially adapted equipment to function fully in programs. In most cases they will bring the devices with them. However, for activities new to the person or for activities with no common adaptations available, makeshift modifications or specially designed equipment may be needed. Equipment should be adapted to provide more independent participation by the person with the disability. For example, adaptations for a person who has difficulty with fine motor skills may include cardholders, large dice or chips, or enlarged paint brush handles. There are many resources available to obtain adapted equipment or assistive technology.

Adaptation to equipment
When fishing, use a chunk of plastic tubing to mount the fishing rod on the wheelchair arm.

Skill requirement. In activities where skills are being taught, such as swimming, canoeing, or dance, an effective way to teach an individual with a disability is to break the activity down into small steps. By breaking the activity down into small tasks, the recreation leader makes only necessary changes in skill requirements. Partial participation is also possible. This means a participant with a disability will be able to participate in a portion of the activity, even if other parts are not feasible for him or her.

Adaptation to skill requirement
In basketball, allow traveling as an alternative for a participant using a wheelchair.

Procedures and/or rules. Recreation leaders are wonderfully notorious for inventing their own activities or modifying popular games to meet the needs of people with varying ages and abilities. By making minor changes in rules or procedures for the individual with a disability or the entire group, success can be achieved by all. For example, when playing tag, a child with asthma can stay on the "safe" space twice as long as the other players to allow a rest period.

Space. Space can be adapted to allow fuller participation in activities. Where accessibility to an area is not feasible, one needs to identify alternate areas where the activity can occur.

Team or group formation. The dynamics of the group or the operation of the group may need to be managed more effectively. For example, if a participant uses a wheelchair and fatigues very easily, but wants to participate in basketball, an adaptation would be having all participants rotate from practicing skills to scrimmaging.

Supports: Additional Staff or Volunteers

If a participant has a need for more intensive staff supervision than usually provided, several strategies may be implemented, including

- ***Assign a one-to-one assistant***. A one-to-one assistant can be a paid or volunteer position who is a support person for the program leader. He or she assists in facilitating the inclusion of the participant with a disability in the program.

- ***Assign an extra staff member***. Instruct them to focus on teaching the basic skills to the participant with a disability. Fade the staff person out as skills are learned.

- ***Develop a "leisure partner" or peer support system***. A leisure partner is a nondisabled peer/participant matched with the participant with a disability who assists as co-player to allow for full participation of the participant with a disability.

- ***Develop a leisure coach system***. Leisure coaches are trained volunteers who teach a leisure or socialization skill to the participant with a disability. Suggestions on where to recruit additional staff for inclusion programs include

  - Universities/colleges
  - Junior and senior high schools
  - Youth groups (e.g., 4-H, Scouts, church groups)
  - Community clubs (e.g., Lions, Legion, Senior Citizens)
  - Advocacy agencies (e.g., Arc, independent living centers)
  - Family, friends, relatives
  - PCAs (personal care attendants)

Step Four: Staff Training

For a smooth and effective inclusion program, all staff (e.g., instructors, leaders, inclusion assistants) must be well-informed. Following are some guidelines and topics for providing staff training so that all staff members feel prepared to work with people of all ability levels.

Adaptation to procedure
Instead of keeping score, the activity may be played for a specific amount of time.

Adaptation to space
A guided nature hike can be moved from a rugged trail to a seldom-used paved back road to allow a wheelchair user to participate.

Adaptation to group formation
Allow for positions to be rotated frequently.

Accommodations and supports can include changing the activity, the equipment, or the staffing in a program.

Anyone who has never made a mistake has never tried anything new.
—Albert Einstein

Well-trained and knowl-
edgable staff is one of the
most important compo-
nents of successful
inclusion.

Staff Training Guidelines

- Training should be ongoing and consistent.

- Training should be conducted with each new program session (e.g., fall, winter, spring, summer).

- Training should be conducted for all program leaders, instructors, and additional staff (if recruited).

- If appropriate and by choice, invite participant and/or parent/guardian to provide additional input into staff training sessions.

- If new staff members are hired in midstream, be sure to educate, train, and orient them to the inclusion process.

Staff Training Topics

Throughout training,
emphasize the value of
diversity.

- Importance of inclusion

- Benefits of inclusion for people with and without disabilities

- Disability awareness activities (e.g., Language and Behavior Awareness Survey; see Chapter 2)

- People-first language

- Simulation/experiential activities (see Appendix C)

- Scenarios—"What would you do in this situation" (see Appendix E)

*We view things not only
from different sides, but
also with different eyes;
we have no wish to find
them alike.*
—Pascal

- Role of the program leader versus the role of the additional staff or volunteers, if recruited (see Appendix F)

- If possible, and if needed, discuss only the important issues of each participant (e.g., handling behaviors, language barriers)

Staff Providing Personal Care Assistance

Some participants with disabilities may require assistance with eating, toileting, or dressing. According to Title II of the Americans With Disabilities Act (Section 35.135), staff members are not required to provide personal care assistance to a participant with a disability unless they provide it as a part of the program to all other participants. If an agency does provide personal services as a part of its programs, then it must also provide it to the participant with a disability (McGovern, 1993, 2000).

*Success is going from
failure to failure without
loss of enthusiasm.*
—Sir Winston Churchill

Some recreation programs have decided that if the participant needs personal care assistance, they will go ahead and provide it in certain circumstances (e.g., a program where young children all need a little assistance changing for swimming or another activity). Some agencies have opted to provide personal care assistance for an extra fee to the participant with a disability. Another approach is to allow a sibling, friend, or the participant's personal care attendant attend the program free and provide the necessary assistance (Stensrud, 1993). Your agency should know its policies on this issue, evaluate each program, and determine how best to apply the policy in a fair and reasonable way.

Nondisabled Peer Orientations

Depending on the individual and the significance of her or his disability, it may be beneficial to orient other participants in a recreation program to disability awareness in general, and to specific needs of the individual being included. Peer orientations are not always desirable or necessary—it depends on the individual and the group. If you conduct a peer orientation, it is always preferable to have the individual with the disability (or parent/guardian, if a minor) share information with the group.

Nondisabled Peer Orientation Topics

Before you conduct a nondisabled peer orientation, permission needs to be granted by the participant and/or parent/guardian. If permission is given, complete the following:

- Invite the participant and/or parent/guardian to provide additional input or ask what they would like to have said. Focus on likenesses more than differences. If the participant has a touch talker, it would be great to orient the peers ahead of time to increase their comfort level.

- Conduct simulation activities (see Appendix C).

- For younger children, read books about specific disabilities, with simulations.

- Give suggestions to other group members on things they can do to help the participant with a disability be included.

- Always allow for questions and discussion time.

Recognizing our common humanity opens all of us to further learning.
—K. E. Eble

Step Five: Program Implementation

At this point all of the previous accommodations and supports should be in place. During the program, be sure to

- Monitor the program by observation.

- Continually structure program activities for social inclusion.

- Meet regularly with program leaders, additional staff, and the participant with a disability to discuss any issues, suggestions, recommendations, or adaptations regarding the program.

- Communicate regularly with parents/guardians, as the participant may express issues with parents/guardians rather than staff.

Step Six: Documentation

Documentation is a part of the overall evaluation of your inclusion efforts in your agency. Have staff document daily the progress of the participant with a disability within the inclusion program. Appendix G contains sample progress documentation forms. Keep a copy of the documentation forms, as this will provide valuable information to new staff members who may work with the participant in future inclusive programs.

Documentation provides the evidence needed to make sound evaluations and thus improve your efforts at inclusion.

The definition of insanity is doing the same thing over and over and expecting different results.
—Benjamin Franklin

Step Seven: Evaluation

At the end of each program session, a summative evaluation should be completed to determine what areas were successful and what areas need improvement. This is something that should be done for *all* recreation programs, not just inclusion programs. The following individuals could complete an evaluation:

- Participant with a disability

- Parent/guardian (if appropriate)

- Program leader/instructor

- Additional staff or volunteers (if recruited)

- Peers without disabilities

Write a summary report from the evaluation results and share it with administrators, staff, board members, potential new program participants, and others who play a large role in your inclusion program. Use the evaluation results to improve your inclusion strategies. Appendix G contains sample evaluation forms.

An overview of the inclusion process is outlined on page 39. At the end of this chapter, a case study (The Case of Anna) provides an example of inclusion in action.

Principles for Structuring Social Integration in Recreation Activities

Leaders can purposefully structure recreation activities to foster social inclusion and positive group interaction.

The inclusion process helps individuals with disabilities to access and to be a part of recreation programs. Yet plenty of research shows that people do not naturally get to know each other in a group situation unless it is structured to encourage the development of positive interactions. This is especially true if some of the group members are noticeably different than the majority, as is the case of many minorities, such as people with disabilities. Coupled with many people's fears of disability, the chances of getting to know other people in a group recreation setting and to develop friendships become remote.

The following principles to structure group recreation activities (from classrooms to teams to camp groups) can help you as a leader to create a situation that will foster positive group interaction and social inclusion (Anderson, 1994). These principles will benefit all participants in the activity, not just the participants with disabilities.

Principle 1
Frequent and consistent opportunities to get acquainted

Structure the recreation activity so that participants can get to know each other.

> **Ideas for Structuring High Acquaintance Potential**
> - Ice breaker activities (e.g., introductions, share favorites)
> - Break into small groups—do activities in small groups
> - Use pairs or partners—have partner introduce other partner to group
> - Mix up groups often
> - Wear nametags

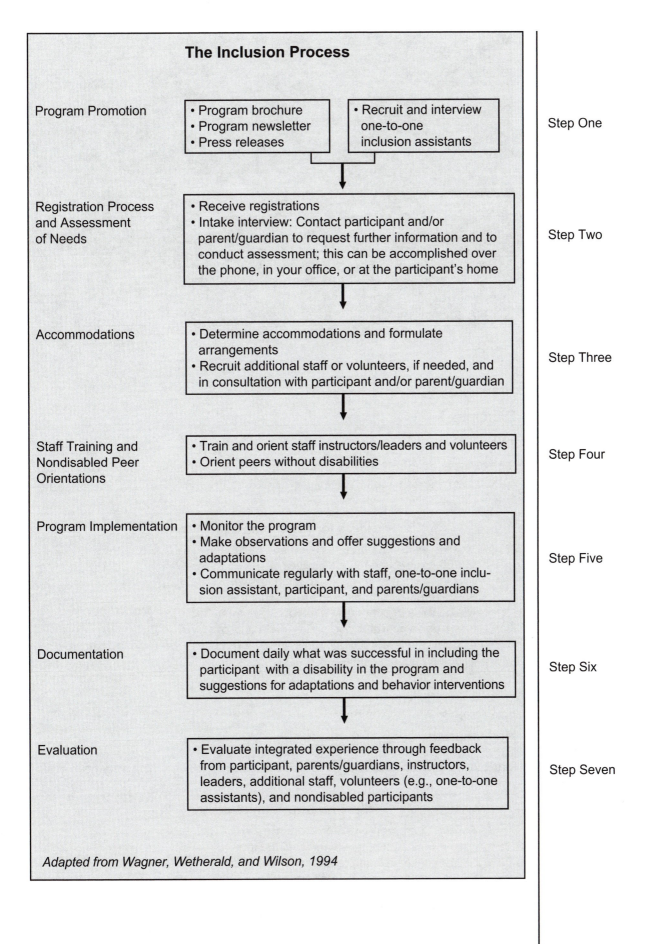

The Inclusion Process

Program Promotion	• Program brochure • Program newsletter • Press releases • Recruit and interview one-to-one inclusion assistants	Step One
Registration Process and Assessment of Needs	• Receive registrations • Intake interview: Contact participant and/or parent/guardian to request further information and to conduct assessment; this can be accomplished over the phone, in your office, or at the participant's home	Step Two
Accommodations	• Determine accommodations and formulate arrangements • Recruit additional staff or volunteers, if needed, and in consultation with participant and/or parent/guardian	Step Three
Staff Training and Nondisabled Peer Orientations	• Train and orient staff instructors/leaders and volunteers • Orient peers without disabilities	Step Four
Program Implementation	• Monitor the program • Make observations and offer suggestions and adaptations • Communicate regularly with staff, one-to-one inclusion assistant, participant, and parents/guardians	Step Five
Documentation	• Document daily what was successful in including the participant with a disability in the program and suggestions for adaptations and behavior interventions	Step Six
Evaluation	• Evaluate integrated experience through feedback from participant, parents/guardians, instructors, leaders, additional staff, volunteers (e.g., one-to-one assistants), and nondisabled participants	Step Seven

Adapted from Wagner, Wetherald, and Wilson, 1994

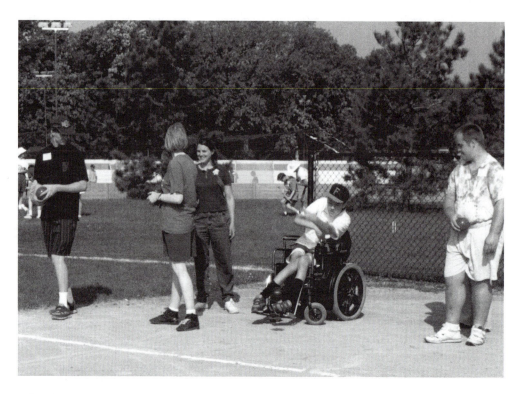

Principle 2
Equal status

Structure the recreation activity and situation so that each participant has equal status in the group, including the participant with a disability.

Ideas for Structuring Equal Status

- Make everyone a part of the decision making
- Mix up groups and responsibilities
- Change format in which information is given
- Ask different group members to demonstrate
- Assign roles in activities—everyone gets to try a role
- Break down activities and skills—everyone can try
- All participants are paying participants—no "special" breaks, no "special" volunteer, no "charity cases"

Principle 3
Mutual goals

Structure the recreation activity so participants perceive they all share a common goal.

Ideas for Structuring Mutual Goals

- Accent teamwork to reinforce equal status
- Leader sets mutual goals and sets the tone
- Leaders verbalize and reinforce mutual goals
- Everyone plays—rotate positions
- Instill spirit, camaraderie
- Give feedback on progress toward goals
- Ask the group to set mutual goals

Courtesy is one of the great human inventions for bridging uncertainty.
—Mary Catherine Bates

Principle 4
Cooperation and interdependence

Structure the recreation activity to include active cooperation and a feeling that each individual's success depends on the successes of the other group members. There are many different ways to structure interdependence (Johnson, Johnson & Holubec, 1991).

Ideas for Structuring Cooperation and Interdependence

- Assign duties or tasks, all are needed to successfully complete the activity
- Use groups to promote team spirit and group identity
- Use team nicknames, T-shirts, other group identifiers
- Keep verbal communication clear
- Use cooperative structure, where each person completes a part of the whole

---

Principle 5
Receiving accurate (not stereotyped) information about the person with a disability

Structure the recreation activity so that all participants receive information about the participant with a disability that is accurate and doesn't perpetuate stereotyped beliefs about the disability.

Ideas for Structuring Accurate Information

- Explain disability or special needs at initial session
- Do ice breaker (similarities vs. differences)
- Assume a can do attitude
- Create an environment of open communication
- Individual determines what should be shared with group
- Draw attention to the participant with a disability when she or he is doing something very well

---

Principle 6
Fair and tolerant norms

Structure the recreation activity so that the situation favors group equality and fairness. Create and reinforce norms that promote fair and caring behavior and tolerance of diversity on the part of the leaders, participants, and spectators.

Ideas for Structuring Egalitarian Norms

- Don't patronize and don't "over help"
- Role model positive, accepting behavior as the leader
- Rotate positions and roles
- Accent positive attributes and skills
- Emphasize teamwork
- Get diverse input from all group members
- Reinforce rules and fairness
- Equal out or balance skill levels

Using these principles a leader can encourage social inclusion and positive group interaction that enriches the recreation experience for *all* participants.

Developing Friendships

*The only way to have a
friend is to be one.*
—Ralph Waldo Emerson

Structuring a recreation activity to promote social integration is an important step in fostering inclusion. Leaders can do even more to help participants develop caring reciprocal relationships. Because many people, whether they have a disability or not, develop and sustain friendships in their leisure, it is important to nurture that development in the programs you lead or manage (Heyne, Schleien & McAvoy, 1993).

Having a clear idea of the main objective of a program will help the leader to develop strategies to make the activity satisfying for everyone. Helping other participants to learn the skills needed to interact with each other will strengthen friendship skills for participants with and without disabilities. For example, help participants to initiate conversation with someone who uses a computer or a touch talker for communication, or help participants to learn some basic sign language, such as "hello" or "how are you?"

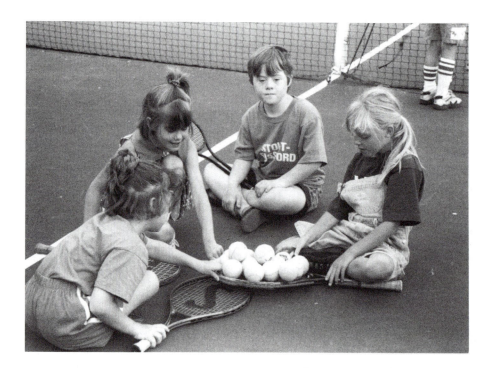

Assignments

Simulations

In Appendix C you will find a series of simulations that can be used in training staff to experience and to develop a better understanding of various types of disabilities.

Mock Intake Interview/Assessment of Needs

In Appendix D you will find an intake interview form and an agency assessment form. With a partner, conduct a mock interview to assess the needs of the participant with a disability who will be participating in your programs.

- Choose one of the participants with a disability that you are planning to include in a recreation program.

- Decide in which program the participant with a disability will be included.

- Decide who will be the recreation provider and who will be the participant with a disability or parent/ guardian (if a minor).

- Once you and your partner have assigned these roles, complete the interview. Remember, these forms are guidelines to help the recreation provider gather the appropriate information needed for an enjoyable experience for everyone in the program.

Scenarios

In Appendix E, you will find six scenarios. With a partner, or with a group of 4–5 people, read each scenario and brainstorm three solutions.

Principles for Structuring Social Inclusion and Positive Group Interaction

Using the principles for structuring social integration and positive group interaction, brainstorm specific actions a group leader could take to put the principles into practice. Build on the examples given in the chapter.

The Inclusion Process: The Case of Anna

Anna is a 10-year-old girl with a developmental disability who registered for a class at the Hometown Recreation Center.

Step One: Program Promotion

The staff at the Hometown Recreation Center reviewed all their brochures, programs, schedules, and other promotional material to look for and change any discriminating statements. They added a statement to all materials that demonstrated their willingness to accommodate everyone in their programs, regardless of ability level. The international symbol of accessibility was displayed next to the statement. Their winter program schedule was sent to every household in Hometown. In addition, they sent copies to local disability and advocacy groups.

Step Two: Registration Process and Assessment of Needs

Anna loved gymnastics. She was glued to the TV whenever gymnastics was on. She pretended to do bar routines on the swing set in the backyard. She begged her mom to buy her a leotard. Due to her disability, her parents had never really thought she could be involved in a sport like gymnastics. When they got the Hometown Recreation Center Winter Program in the mail, they were surprised and pleased to see the welcoming statements and openness to have children of all abilities in their programs. The parents decided to try Anna in one of the gymnastics classes, despite their reservations, because Anna was so interested. They filled out the registration form in the winter schedule. On the form, they checked the question that asked if Anna had any specific accommodations or needs to participate.

When Gina, the gymnastics instructor, got the winter class registration forms, she called Anna's family and invited them in for a tour and orientation to the class. During the tour, Gina interviewed Anna and her parents to see what kind of needs Anna would have to participate fully in the gymnastics program. Anna's parents informed Gina that, until this year, Anna had been in a segregated classroom at school and her social skills weren't at the level of her peers. She had never participated in a recreation center class before, and it took her a while to learn new things. Anna was very quiet and shy during the tour, but her parents informed Gina that she had difficulty taking turns in groups and got loud and excitable at times. Gina asked the parents if Anna had any medical needs she should be aware of. Gina encouraged Anna and her parents to ask any questions they had about the program at any time.

Step Three: Accommodations and Supports

Gina shared with Anna and her parents some ideas she had on how to best include Anna in the beginning gymnastics class. Together with the parents and Anna, Gina decided on the following supports and accommodations for Anna:

- Anna would observe some of the class sessions with her parents so she would have an awareness of what the classes were like.
- Gina would have Anna register in the beginning class with other girls about her age. Because it was a beginning class, Gina would break down the skills being taught into small steps so that they could be more easily learned by Anna as well as the other girls.
- Before including Anna in the class, and with Anna and her parents' permission, Gina would inform the other girls that Anna would be joining the class. She would let them know that Anna had a disability, but would primarily focus on how much she is like them versus how she is different. She would let them ask any questions they had about disability issues. Anna's mom would come to that class, if she had time, and help to answer questions.
- Gina would get two or three of the other girls in the class to volunteer to be leisure partners for Anna. They would take turns helping Anna to understand the directions given and anything else to help her be included in the class session. Gina would help the girls learn their role as a leisure partner, making sure they do not "over help" Anna. As Anna becomes more accustomed to the class, the girls would need to help her less. If it appeared that Anna needed more help than the leisure partners and Gina could give her, then Gina would have another staff member assigned to assist her with the class. With two instructors, there would be less waiting time in line, and less chance for Anna to show poor behavior.
- Gina and other girls in the class would role model good social skills. Gina would give Anna praise when she waited in line for her turn well. If Anna was disruptive during the class, she would be expected to change her behavior when she was asked. If not, Gina would use the same policy with Anna that the Center used with any disruptive behavior.
- Because Anna had no physical or mobility impairments, it was not necessary to use adapted equipment or other devices. Gina identified with Anna and her parents that most of the supports needed were in the social and learning areas of the class sessions.

Step Four: Staff Training and Nondisabled Peer Orientations

Prior to the beginning of the winter session, the Hometown Recreation Center Director had conducted staff training sessions for all new staff and any staff who needed to refresh their orientation. An important part of the staff training was the area of inclusion. Gina knew that if she needed an additional staff member to assist her in beginner gymnastics class, that person would have an awareness of inclusion and disability issues. Gina would only need to update him or her on Anna's particular needs.

Because Anna's social skills were not at the level of her peers, Gina and Anna's parents decided to orient the other girls in the class to Anna's disability. The orientation would help the girls understand why Anna did not yet know how to wait her turn well or why she would sometimes yell loudly and get overly excited. By understanding Anna's behavior, the other girls could help her learn, instead of teasing her or being afraid of her. Gina would give the girls suggestions on things they could do to include Anna in the gymnastics activities. For example, Gina would suggest that the other girls waiting in line by Anna talk to her about things they like and find out what kinds of things Anna likes.

Step Five: Program Implementation

Gina implemented the planned inclusion program for Anna. She communicated with Anna's mom or dad when they dropped her off or picked her up on how Anna was doing in the class. They communicated with Gina on how Anna looked forward to the class times each week. Gina observed how the other girls were interacting with Anna. The three leisure partners were given an orientation and were helping Anna in the class sessions. Gina communicated frequently with the girls to see how being a leisure partner was going for them. Gina observed Anna's behavior in class sessions. She observed and learned what things seem to get Anna overly excited and was able to avoid those situations. Anna talked with other girls while waiting turns. She did not show any disruptive behavior and was able to take turns well. A few times, Gina was unable to teach her classes. The staff members who filled in for Gina were well-informed on inclusion and on Anna's needs, so there were no problems.

Step Six: Documentation

At the beginning of the gymnastics program, Gina was given a documentation form. It was her responsibility to document daily on Anna's progress. She documented what strategies and/or adaptations she used to include Anna in the gymnastics program. For example, Gina documented how positive feedback was used with Anna for behavior management, how Anna's peers were working out as leisure partners, how positive role modeling was having an effect on Anna, how at times, she used pictures of skills to help Anna learn the skills better. The information provided on the documentation forms was specific and concrete, so future staff members could use it when Anna moved to the next level or to a different program.

Step Seven: Evaluation

At the end of the winter session of gymnastics at the Hometown Recreation Center, Gina had the girls in her beginner gymnastics class give her some feedback on how the session went using a written evaluation form. She also got written and verbal feedback from the parents of the girls in the session and from the additional staff who were involved. The evaluation information helped Gina determine if the program had been successful for all who were involved, as well as areas that needed improvement. Gina compiled the results into a simple evaluation report, including a summary of the daily documentation notes. She shared the evaluation report with the Hometown Recreation Director. The Director shared the information with her Board of Directors, and with potential new participants who asked about the Hometown Recreation Center programs. The evaluation report helped the Center to get more support for inclusion efforts in their programs.

Chapter 5

What Are the Administrative Concerns With Inclusion?

Administrators in the parks and recreation field need to consider the following concerns when planning and implementing inclusive recreation programs. Without administrative support inclusion will not prosper at any agency. Efforts at the administrative level must support and complement efforts at the individual and program level.

Mission and Philosophy

To create accessible programs, services, and facilities, an agency needs to develop an inclusive mission and philosophy. The philosophy should be articulated clearly, in writing and as philosophical tenets, so that all staff members at an agency understand the basic beliefs that guide their organization. Within this philosophy a commitment must be made to serve everyone, regardless of ability. The expression of this philosophy results in the mission statement. This is a statement of purpose for the agency.

- The mission statement reflects the vision and values that direct an agency and empowers and guides an agency to achieve its goals and objectives.

- The mission statement and its philosophical tenets become the basis for making decisions in the midst of circumstances that affect an agency.

- The mission statement may need to be rewritten to eliminate discriminatory practices if they exist.

Examples of Inclusive and Nondiscriminatory Mission Statements

The mission of Bismarck Parks and Recreation District is to promote broad-based recreation opportunities to improve the quality of life for the citizens of Bismarck and its visitors.
- To increase and enhance the recreational opportunities for all ages, stages, and abilities
- To increase public awareness as to the benefits of and participation in parks and recreation
- To promote professionalism in the delivery of parks and recreation services
- To increase the understanding of the contributions made by parks and recreation to the economy and economic development

The mission of Grafton Parks and Recreation District is to promote recreational and leisure opportunities for all individuals to enrich their quality of life.

Our mission [Wilderness Inquiry] is to use outdoor experiences as a means to bring people together. Wilderness Inquiry provides experiences that combine people with and without disabilities from diverse backgrounds. Our trips are shared cooperative adventures that combine the strength and positive energy of all members in the group.

The mission of Pine to Prairie Girl Scouts is to inspire in all girls the highest ideals of character, conduct, patriotism, and service that they may become happy and resourceful citizens.

What lies behind us and what lies before us are tiny matters compared to what lies within us.
—Oliver Wendell Holmes

The *mission statement* must clearly articulate that all people, including people with disabilities, are welcomed and served by your agency.

The Pine to Prairie Girl Scout Council has addressed administrative support for inclusion. Its administrative staff has received training on inclusion. Its mission statement, policies, and procedures were examined and modified to reflect inclusion. Its field training for troop leaders was revised to address inclusion needs. It sought additional funding for inclusion efforts. It actively sought partnerships with disability organizations such as the Arc. This exemplary administrative support has ensured that the Pine to Prairie Girl Scout Council is a welcoming, accessible agency.

Constant self-evaluation ensures that community needs are being met in the most inclusive manner.

We are what we repeatedly do. Excellence, then, is not an act, but a habit.
—Aristotle

Self-Evaluation

Conducting a self-evaluation of programs, services, policies, and procedures within the agency will assist in determining what supports and accommodations will be essential to serving persons with disabilities. Self-evaluation was also discussed in Chapter 3, in relation to meeting the mandate of the ADA. Unfortunately, some agencies have completed the required self-evaluation, filed it away, and done little with it once the requirement was met. To evolve to a truly inclusive agency, constant self-evaluation must occur.

When conducting the self-evaluation to develop and implement programs, services, policies, and procedures, recreation and leisure service providers need to consider the following:

- Review interest survey results, program evaluations, and community recommendations annually.

- Conduct focus groups where consumers with and without disabilities, parents, recreation/leisure service providers, human service providers, and other interested individuals meet to evaluate the needs of the community as to what recreation programs and services are available.

- Survey community residents with disabilities to assure their recreational needs are being met.

- Evaluate the programs you offer. Are some cooperative in nature? Do they encourage social interaction? Can friendships be developed? Are they fun, functional, and age-appropriate?

- Evaluate the diversity of activities you offer. Are there a variety of recreational programs to choose from? Are there programs that meet the needs of everyone in their community? Are there other agencies with which you can collaborate to more effectively meet community needs?

- Evaluate policies and procedures of the agency to assure that they reflect the mission. It is imperative to emphasize to the staff, through ongoing and consistent training, the need to recognize the individuality of their consumers.

- Provide leisure opportunities that are personally satisfying in respect to the changing needs, interests, and abilities of the population. Leisure opportunities should be directed at developing the whole self and providing each person with autonomy, self-determination, and respect.

Administrative Support

For an agency to be truly welcoming to all people, all employees must believe in an inclusive philosophy. An excellent way to describe total agency commitment to an inclusive philosophy is " top-down, bottom-up."

- Executive directors, board members, and others who head the agency must believe in an inclusive philosophy and support the goals of the mission.

- Support for inclusion must also come from full-time employees, part-time employees, and even volunteers. It must come from program specialists to instructors to maintenance staff.

Having this support filtered down from the top and up from the bottom will create a welcoming and user-friendly environment for all consumers.

Consumer Input

To better serve persons with disabilities of all ages, it is imperative to include their input during the planning, implementation, and evaluation of inclusive services.

- Individuals with disabilities are an excellent resource to use when examining physical accessibility as well as program accessibility.

- Consumer input is needed to evaluate the effectiveness of the changes the agency has made.

- Consumers with disabilities are speaking from experience. They know and understand directly what the barriers are and how people with disabilities want and should be treated.

- Independent living centers, Arcs, and other advocacy organizations are good ways to make contact with people with disabilities.

Never doubt that a small group of thoughtful, committed citizens can change the world; indeed, it is the only thing that ever has.
—Margaret Mead

Advisory Committee Development

Develop an advisory committee that specifically addresses the recreation and leisure needs of persons with disabilities. This advisory board could be made up of consumers with varying types of disabilities, parents, advocacy groups, therapeutic recreation specialists, school personnel, the general public, and other interested individuals who advocate for people with disabilities.

Sample Objectives of Advisory Committee

To bring together individuals and agencies to facilitate community recreation opportunities for people with disabilities through networking, advocacy, and action

To serve as a resource to individuals with and without disabilities, and to advise leisure service providers on methods to achieve physical and program access within community settings

To promote public awareness about the value and availability of recreation opportunities in community settings through dissemination of information

To develop a working relationship with a variety of community leisure service agencies to effect greater opportunities for community recreation participation

Schleien, Ray, and Green (1997)

Safety and Liability

There is a myth of an increase in liability when children or adults with disabilities participate in recreation programs. Fear of injury and a resulting lawsuit can make agencies cautious and even reluctant to promote inclusion. In reality, providing services to people with disabilities has no more risk than providing services to any program participant. In fact, an agency is more at risk from a lawsuit if it doesn't provide services than if it does. Good planning and quality services are the keys to reduced liability.

An agency is more at risk from a lawsuit if it doesn't provide inclusive services than if it does.

You can't roll up your sleeves and get to work if you're still wringing your hands.
—Old Proverb

Following are four "safety tasks" for inclusion programmers (Schleien, McAvoy, Lais & Rynders, 1993):

1. Reduce unnecessary risk through adequate training and proper program design.
2. Convince the sponsoring agency that the proposed program is not unreasonably risky.
3. Convince participants, parents, and guardians that the program is safe.
4. Conduct the program in such a way that the probability of an accident is low.

Schleien, McAvoy, Lais, and Rynders (1993) identified the following steps to assist in a safe, injury-free program and to minimize the likelihood of liability suits:

1. Thorough program planning with documents addressing
   - Participant permission and registration forms
   - Records of staff qualifications and training
   - Medical information forms
   - Procedures for responding to accidents
   - Records of program and staff evaluations
2. Appropriate numbers of qualified staff members (with appropriate skills/ competencies for activity).
   - The ratio of staff-to-participants varies depending on the program and skill level of the participants
   - The proportion of people with disabilities to people without disabilities should reflect the natural proportion of people with disabilities in society—about 1 in 5
   - "Qualified staff" means that the staff member has the skills for the recreation activity and the skills to work with groups of varying abilities, in addition to other needed competencies

A "qualified staff" member has
- Skills for the recreation activity
- Skills to work with groups of varying abilities
- Safety skills and other basic competencies
- Good judgment

3. The recreation activity and the location of the activity must be appropriate for participants and their skill levels.
4. Develop a sense of community and an atmosphere of self-responsibility.
5. Inform participants of potential risks; be sure they understand the risks to encourage self-responsibility.
6. Supervision is critical for a safe program. General responsibilities of the staff and agency to provide safe opportunities for all participants include the following:
   - Operate facilities that adhere to appropriate standards of safety available to children, youth, and adults.
   - Equipment must be appropriate for the activity and the participants' skill level and must be properly maintained.
   - Staff members must be trained in appropriate safety techniques and emergency recreation procedures, which are standardized and well-documented.
   - Staff members must be trained to provide programs appropriate to skill levels and capabilities of participants under supervision.
7. Staff members must exercise good judgment in using facilities and program components.

Funding

Funding is always a concern for administrators. Finding and maintaining the funds to provide inclusive recreation services requires a creative mind. Remember that providing inclusive services is less costly in the long run than providing special segregated programs. Following are some tips on maximizing funding potential for your agency.

- Through networking, the costs of running programs may be diminished. The ability to utilize other staff and/or facilities decreases the cost of inclusion and increases the effectiveness of inclusive programming. Sharing resources and expertise between agencies reduces duplication and increases efficiency and quality.

- Develop a committee that directly seeks funding from interest groups, corporate foundations, and state and federal grants that fund specifically for persons with disabilities, collaborative programs, and diversity programs.

- Pursuing funds through donations and/or corporate foundations is enhanced when programs are designed for utilization by the entire community, and when collaboration between agencies is strong.

- Federal grants are available from the U.S. Department of Education, Office of Special Education and Rehabilitative Services to upgrade personnel development or develop innovative programs. The Catalog of Federal Domestic Assistance, available online (http://www.cfda.gov) or at any city or university library, contains announcements about federal grant competitions.

- For physical accessibility, capital grants may be pursued through the U.S. Department of Transportation (http://www.dot.gov).

- State Developmental Disabilities Councils receive federal block grants to disperse at the state level to improve services for people with developmental disabilities. To contact your state Developmental Disability Council, access these websites: The National Association of Developmental Disabilities Councils (http://www.naddc.org) or the Consortium of Developmental Disabilities Councils (http://www.cddc.com).

- State professional associations, such as the state Recreation and Parks Association, often offer conferences or workshops on effective grant writing. Also, many advocacy groups, such as the Arc or independent living centers, would be excellent resources for technical assistance with grant writing, as well as collaboration on a program proposal.

Sharing resources and expertise across agencies not only is cost-effective but also increases the quality of services.

Although grants and other external funds are an effective way to initiate efforts at inclusion, agencies should plan for inclusion costs to be part of their ongoing operating budget in the future.

A Few Tips on Writing Effective Grants

- Clearly present your request
- Describe your agency's qualifications and strengths
- Document the needs well—present them as opportunities rather than problems
- Set measurable objectives
- Have a clear evaluation plan
- Clearly delineate the costs for which you seek funding
- Show evidence of broad community support for your request

Thunder is good, thunder is impressive, but it is lightning that does the work.
—Mark Twain

Staff

Providing staff properly trained in working and interacting with people with disabilities concerns some administrators. Working with people with disabilities does not take anyone "special"; rather, it takes someone who has the attitude of accepting and understanding the diverse needs and abilities of participants. Also, recreation agencies should strive to hire staff members who have disabilities as well.

The following are a few ideas an administrator may want to keep in mind for their staff. These suggestions will assist the employer and new staff in developing a professional relationship as they understand the mission and philosophy of the agency.

Job Description

The first place an employer is able to assert the importance of being able to include persons with disabilities into community programs is the job description. The job description for community recreation professionals should focus on having an understanding of the needs of people with disabilities and the willingness to provide accessible leisure services to community members. This should be in writing.

Hiring

When hiring new staff, the agency should express their mission and philosophy clearly. Emphasize the importance of inclusion of *all* people, which includes people with disabilities. If appropriate, ask the person if they have experience or knowledge in working with people with disabilities. Also, ask if they are comfortable in having a person with a disability in their program.

A positive, open attitude about including people with disabilities in programs and services is a critical factor to assess when hiring new staff.

Lacking experience or knowledge in working with people with disabilities should not be the factor that determines whether or not an applicant gets the job. More important is an applicant's attitude toward inclusion and diversity. A positive, open attitude is crucial in an agency that promotes accessibility. It should, however, help the employer to identify the fears and concerns the individual may have along with developing an understanding of the importance of serving everybody on an individual basis.

Training

Training of existing staff to provide adaptations for individuals with disabilities may mean that less specialized staff needs to be hired or recruited. This can be done through in-service training programs for both staff and volunteers. The training should be ongoing, comprehensive and relevant to the inclusion process and persons with disabilities. Staff training for inclusion was discussed in Chapter 4.

Marketing

An often-heard comment from recreation service providers is "there aren't people with disabilities in our community" or "people with disabilities don't come to our programs." If an agency has a history of inaccessible programs and facilities, people with disabilities probably have stopped coming or have never tried to be a participant. Marketing of inclusive recreation programs is an important aspect in serving the entire community.

- First, develop a marketing plan to determine the course of action that will be taken.

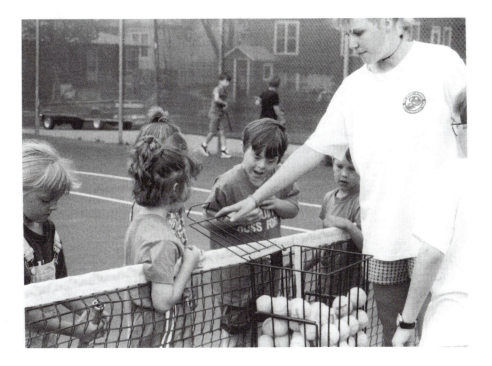

All staff at your agency are the "advertisers" of your program's mission and values on inclusion. The person who answers the phone, the janitor—they all create the impression that your agency provides welcoming services.

- Identify the audience to whom your agency's services are promoted.

- The plan should identify individuals and agencies that provide social, education, and health services to persons with disabilities, including a list of consumers with disabilities in your community.

- Make contact with potential users to persuade them to become active users through a variety of media (e.g., brochures, flyers, advertisements in local newspapers, personal phone calls). If the potential user has an impairment that makes communication difficult, initially communicate through parents, friends, or guardians. Be sure the International Symbol of Access is clearly displayed on all media.

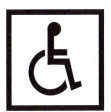

- You may need to describe the modifications and adaptations that you will use to accommodate the individual's needs.

- Statements of nondiscrimination that welcome participants of all abilities sound friendly, sensitive, and inviting to all potential participants of the leisure experience and help to market programs. Here is an example from the Eden Prairie Parks, Recreation, and Natural Resource Department brochure:

    The city of Eden Prairie is committed to providing reasonable accommodations and accessibility to all our residents. If you require a sign language interpreter or assistance to register or participate, please contact our Therapeutic Recreation Coordinator at 952–949-8452 or TTY: 952–949-8399 to ensure that we meet your accessibility needs. Prior contact of three weeks is preferred.

- Word-of-mouth is a powerful marketing tool. If one person with a disability has a positive experience at your agency, the word will spread. Remember, however, that a negative experience will have the same effect.

- How written material is presented in promotional material is a key factor for people with and without disabilities to understand the information.

┌───┐
│   │
│   Suggestions for Preparing Accessible Information   │
│   │
│   •   Provide information on audiotape, videotape, computer disk, or webpage │
│   •   Use bold lettering to emphasize important information │
│   •   Provide information in large print   │
│   •   Use short, to the point sentences   │
│   •   Provide pictures with written information   │
│   •   Block off or highlight key information   │
│   •   Provide the name and phone number of a contact person │
│   │
└───┘

Traits of a Quality Program

What constitutes a quality inclusive recreation program for a person with a disability? Are there signs with which a consumer with a disability or parent/guardian can identify? Are there traits that service providers can strive to include in their programs? Rynders and Schelien (1991) have developed the following list of quality indicators in community recreation services, focusing on the level of commitment to inclusion.

Administration

- Mission statement/philosophy reflects belief in inclusion.

- Hiring criteria for staff—give credit for education and/or experience reflecting inclusion.

- Adherence to laws and legislation pertaining to serving persons with disabilities in least restrictive recreation environment.

- Staff training priorities emphasize continuing education in topical areas, such as innovations and techniques in inclusion and use of community-based consultants.

- Documentation of inclusive services/interventions provided and the effects on participants recorded systematically.

Nature of Program

- Offers inclusive programs or segregated–integrated programs (allows for choice).

- Provides flexible programs that allow for ongoing modifications/adaptations (allows for partial participation, if needed).

- Program goals reflect an inclusion emphasis (e.g., heterogeneous activity provisions, friend-oriented interaction modes).

Activities

- Age-appropriate.

- Functional and lifelong.

- Allow for participant choice.

- Mix of individualistic, cooperative, and competitive styles.

Whatever you can do, or dream, you can begin it. Boldness has genius, power and magic in it.
—Goethe

Examples of Activities
Individualistic style
Aerobics
Cooperative style
Drama activities
Competitive style
Team sports

- Generalizable across time and environments.

- Allow for personal challenge (dignity and risk).

Environmental/Logistical Considerations

- Physically accessible and easily allow for modifications.

- Offered activities are at convenient and appropriate times for those whom program serves.

- Cost is reasonable and sponsorships are available.

Techniques and Methods

- Ongoing assessment and evaluation of participants' leisure needs, preferences, skills, and enjoyment.

- Inclusion of parents/guardians and consumers with disabilities in assessments and evaluations.

- Inclusion techniques such as task analysis, environmental analysis, partial participation, and companionship training utilized regularly.

- Ongoing program evaluation to make needed adaptations and modifications.

- Appropriate use of paid (or preferably unpaid) leisure partners (e.g., friends, peers).

Assignment

Equal Opportunity Recreation Provider

Being an equal opportunity recreation provider involves everyone in your agency, from the board of directors and administration to the leaders and instructors in programs to the maintenance staff.

To identify if you are an equal opportunity recreation provider, answer the statements on the following survey. If you answer *yes* to all the statements, you are an equal opportunity recreation provider. If you answered *no* to any of the statements, then barriers to participation that can limit some individuals from being included in typical general recreation opportunities exist. For the questions you answered *no*, identify ways your agency can change to be more inclusive of all people. What action steps will you or your agency initiate to provide a full inclusive environment?

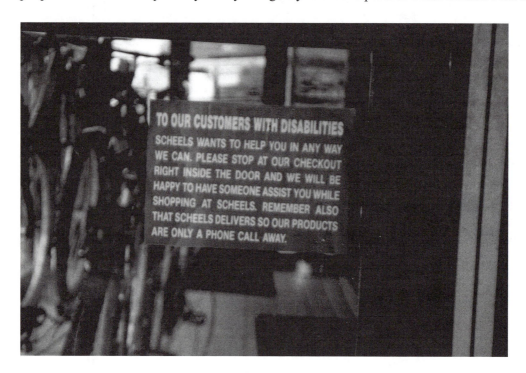

Are You An Equal Opportunity Recreation Provider?

Does your agency...

1. Consult with persons who have different abilities to determine their recreation needs?   yes   no

2. Plan inclusive programs to meet the identified interests and needs of people who have differing abilities?   yes   no

3. Meet with parents to plan inclusive opportunities for children and youth receiving special education services and supports?   yes   no

4. Provide all programs in barrier-free facilities?   yes   no

5. Promote your programs as being inclusive of all persons who have a variety of abilities?   yes   no

6. Plan purchases of new recreation equipment that can be used by participants with a variety of abilities?   yes   no

7. Assist individuals to participate as independently as possible in all phases of recreation programs?   yes   no

8. Provide volunteer support for persons who need assistance to participate?   yes   no

9. Focus on each individual's abilities, needs, and preferences rather than his or her disabilities?   yes   no

10. Identify initiatives in your community recreation plan to address individual needs of all people and to provide accessible inclusive programs, services, and facilities?   yes   no

Burkhour (1992)

Chapter 6

What Is Networking?

Networking is the process of establishing and maintaining communication with professionals and consumers from a variety of backgrounds that have a common vision about community leisure services. This cooperative relationship occurs between individuals from various professional disciplines, consumers, agencies, or organizations. They benefit from pooling information, resources, and technical assistance. The primary reason for networking by two or more agencies is to better meet the needs of consumers. The consumer is the center of the partnership. Through networking, agencies can serve a greater number of individuals with disabilities.

What Are the Benefits of Networking?

- Agencies can increase internal resources by adding the specialized skills of staff that work with the other agencies with which they network. For example, a human service agency can provide guidance and information regarding the special needs of people with disabilities who participate in inclusive community recreation programs. Leisure service professionals provide expertise in planning, teaching, and leading recreation activities as well as facilities and equipment. Networking enriches the internal resources of both agencies.

- Staff within the network may be able to assist other agencies during their periods of peak use, leading to higher quality services (i.e., services that best meet customers' needs) and improved resource utilization.

- Individuals with disabilities receive better services due to enhanced facilities and programs offered within the network. When networking professionals can focus on and use the strengths of each individual within the network, greater success is achieved by all.

- Networking requires communication that increases the flow of information between and within the organizations in the network. For example, a local therapeutic recreation specialist in a hospital may prepare a discharge plan with an individual with a disability and (with appropriate permission) share that plan with a community recreation professional. With this increased communication, it is more likely that the individual with the disability will receive better services. The community recreation professional will be aware of the needs of the individual and can consult with the hospital therapeutic recreation specialist for assistance.

- The networking process enables professionals to be informed and to keep peers informed within and outside their respective fields. Networks provide more diverse programs, better facilities, and a variety of trained professionals who collaborate to provide better overall services to improve the quality of life of the individuals they serve.

- Networks share a common vision of inclusive recreation. This vision creates a rippling effect for advocacy for the rights of people with disabilities. No longer is it just the parents or the advocacy groups trying to improve services—it is all agencies in the network.

We cannot live for ourselves alone. Our lives are connected by a thousand invisible threads, and along these sympathetic fibers, our actions run as causes and return to us as results.
—Herman Melville

Benefits of Networking
- Enhanced services
- Improved communication
- Greater information flow
- Increased diversity
- Advocacy rippling effect

What Are the Elements of Networking?

Networking can occur within and between agencies or organizations. Intraorganizational networking refers to a series of networks that operate within an organization for a shared goal to improve the organization. Interorganizational networks share common goals or issues. Whether internal or community-wide, several elements make a network successful.

Keys to Effective Networking
- Common vision
- Communication
- Compromise (win–win)
- Commitment
- Consumer involvement by people with disabilities
- Clarity (roles, authority)

- ***Decide if you have enough in common to start a partnership***. Everyone involved in the network must share a common vision. Networking combines missions through mutually agreed on goals and objectives for agencies and individual customers. Everyone must be committed to the shared vision and motivated to accomplish it.

- ***Evaluate the strengths and weaknesses of all individuals involved in the network***. This allows for increased success by supplementing the weaknesses and complementing the strengths. An understanding that networks are long-term relationships is necessary to overcome short-term failures. Networks may not achieve immediate goals, but they will eventually provide positive results.

- ***Compromise***. Individuals within the network should take risks without anticipating rejection. Others need to be receptive to new ideas. Within the network, there may be many differing philosophies. Always search for win–win solutions.

To affect the quality of the day, that is the highest of arts.
—Henry David Thoreau

- ***Communicate***. Remain in touch with those involved—it is the key to success. Communication increases motivation, shares important information regarding progress toward the goal, and provides assistance when facing a difficult task. Continued communication with individuals with disabilities promotes motivated employees and provides information regarding the consumers' satisfaction and views. Everyone in the partnership or network must know how much authority they have in representing their agency and what level of involvement is desired or needed.

What Can I Do to Promote Networking and Collaboration?

- Keep an open mind.
- Satisfy your need for information—ask questions, seek clarification.
- Expand your sources of support and information—bring more people into the network.
- Be responsible—follow through on your part of the partnership.
- Provide information and offer suggestions.
- Know your limits and when to ask for help.
- Recognize the efforts of others—give feedback.
- Value and act on the expertise of others in the network.
- Obtain training and information that will increase your skills.
- Listen.
- Remember why you are collaborating—keep foremost in your mind and efforts the people with disabilities whom you are helping to lead more satisfying, enriched lives through inclusive recreation.

Networks are comprised of individuals—each has a part in making the network successful.

Model Collaborative Programs for Inclusive Recreation

The following programs are resources to enlarge your network. These agencies and organizations have developed exemplary inclusive recreation programs. Most have been able to achieve their success through partnerships and networking.

Bismarck Parks and Recreation District and Bismarck Public Schools, Bismarck, ND

Bismarck Parks and Recreation and Bismarck Public Schools combined their summer programs as a collaborative educational and community recreational program. The 10-week summer program is for children in grades K–6 and is provided in 12 neighborhood elementary schools and parks throughout Bismarck. The inclusion of children with disabilities is an integral part of the program. As a result of this partnership, and its success with inclusion, Bismarck Parks and Recreation District has now added a full-time CTRS to its staff to foster even more inclusion across all their programs.

For more information, contact:
Steve Neu, CPRP
701–222–6455
http://www.bisparks.org

Eden Prairie Parks, Recreation, and Natural Resources Department, Eden Prairie, MN

The city of Eden Prairie's Adaptive Recreation Program serves as a model for inclusion of people with disabilities into Eden Prairie's parks and recreation opportunities. Eden Prairie is part of a four-city cooperative that promotes inclusive recreation, community education, and related services for people with disabilities. The other cities in the cooperative are Bloomington, Edina, and Richfield. A therapeutic recreation specialist coordinates Eden Prairie's Adaptive Recreation Program. The mission of the program is to provide and enhance access in recreation and leisure services for individuals with disabilities and to provide resources, education, and support to those who live, work, and play in Eden Prairie. It is not just adaptive programming anymore. Inclusion opportunities through Eden Prairie's Adaptive Recreation Program continue to grow dramatically each year. Over 200 people with disabilities are included in all aspects of Eden Prairie's recreation programs. Inclusion plays a large role in all recreation programs offered by the agency, and is viewed positively by all involved—staff, parents, and people with disabilities.

As for adaptive programming, it continues to exist on an as needed basis. Adaptive programs are designed to teach the skills needed (e.g., physical, social, cognitive) for a person with a disability to then move on to the same program in an inclusive setting. Basically, adaptive programs are developed and implemented with the intention of being short-term and a stepping stone to inclusive recreation programs. Often, people with disabilities do not need adaptive programming and benefit much more by participating in inclusive recreation settings.

For more information, contact:
Carla Brown Kress, CTRS
952–949–8442
http://www.edenprairie.org

Snowflakes are one of nature's most fragile things, but just look what they can do when they stick together.
—Verna M. Kelly

It's amazing what you can accomplish if you do not care who gets the credit.
—Harry S. Truman

Turtle River State Park and Options Independent Living Center, Arvilla, ND and East Grand Forks, MN

Turtle River State Park, situated in the Red River Valley, offers an array of outdoor recreation opportunities, exhibits and programming. In a partnership with Options Independent Living Center, the park staff and people with disabilities have assessed the park and its programs for accessibility. Together they have developed and implemented plans to make this state park a welcoming, accessible recreation attraction.

For more information, contact:
Turtle River State Park
North Dakota Parks and Recreation Department
701–594–4445
http://www.ndparks.com/TRSP.htm

A willingness to offer full participation to all its people is in some sense the criterion of a good society.
—Mary Catherine Bateson

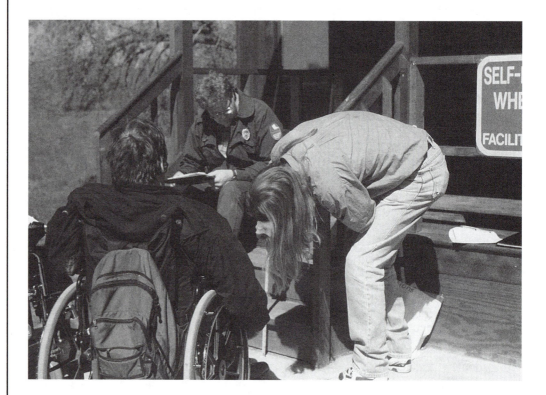

Grand Forks Cooperative Inclusion Program, Grand Forks, ND

Four agencies providing recreation services—the Grand Forks Park District, the Grand Forks YMCA Family Center, the LISTEN Social Drop-In Center, and Red River Valley Gymnastics—teamed up for the Cooperative Inclusion Program. The agencies developed and submitted a grant proposal to a nonprofit foundation, which was funded. All four agencies shared a full-time therapeutic recreation specialist, who worked with inclusion of people with disabilities at the agencies. The therapeutic recreation specialist took a lead role in staff training, self-evaluation, and accessibility planning, and provision of technical assistance with staff members as they included people of all ability levels in programs and activities offered by all four agencies. By sharing a full-time therapeutic recreation specialist, all agencies were able to move more quickly toward the provision of inclusive programming.

For more information, contact:
Grand Forks Park District
701–746–2750
http://www.gfparks.org

Pine to Prairie Girl Scout Council and Arc Upper Valley, Grand Forks, ND

Pine to Prairie Girl Scout Council stretches from eastern North Dakota to western Minnesota. Its mission is to provide opportunities for girls of all abilities to develop their full potential. The Arc Upper Valley is an advocacy and resource center, helping people with disabilities to achieve full inclusion in their communities in all aspects of their lives. These two agencies have collaborated to ensure that the opportunities provided by the Girl Scouts are fully accessible to girls of all abilities. Through sharing of their resources and expertise, these two agencies have increased the number of girls with disabilities in neighborhood Girl Scout Troops across the area.

For more information, contact:
Pine to Prairie Girl Scout Council
701–772–6679
http://www.girlscoutsptpc.org

Wilderness Inquiry, Minneapolis, MN

Wilderness Inquiry is a nonprofit organization whose mission is to provide outdoor adventure experiences around the world to people of all abilities. Since 1978 its successes have made it a model program on inclusion. It enjoys many partnerships with other agencies, such as the U.S. Forest Service, the National Park Service, and the Wilderness Society. Wilderness Inquiry provides inclusive outdoor trips to areas such as the Boundary Waters Canoe Area Wilderness, Yellowstone National Park, and the Florida Everglades. Wilderness Inquiry believes that no barrier to inclusion is insurmountable and the most powerful way to eliminate barriers is through attitude and group interaction. Wilderness Inquiry does not believe that wild areas should be paved to be made accessible. Rather, the group must work together to achieve access so that everyone, regardless of ability, can enjoy our beautiful wilderness areas.

For more information, contact:
Greg Lais, Executive Director
800–728–0719 (voice or TTY)
http://www.wildernessinquiry.org

The wilderness can be for anyone—no matter what background, abilities, or other circumstances they may have.
—Wilderness Inquiry participant

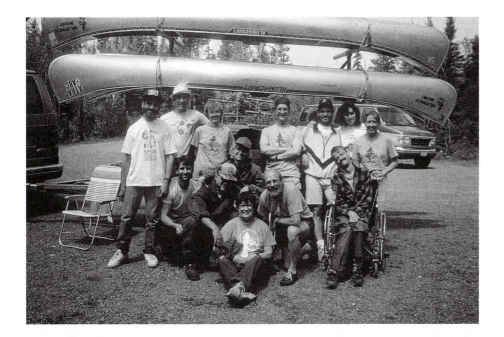

This trip renewed my respect and love for the environment as well as my conviction that contact with the natural elements brings out the very best in people.
—Wilderness Inquiry participant

Assignment

Assess Your Collaborative Skills

Collaboration brings together people from diverse backgrounds and interests so they may share knowledge, skills, and resources. For a collaborative partnership to function, you must know and use small group interpersonal skills. Take a few moments to assess your own collaborative skills (Thousand & Villa, 1992).

Review your self-assessment. Put an asterik (*) by those skills you scored 2 or below on and would like to improve to become a more effective collaborating partner. Develop a personal action plan to improve and put these skills into use.

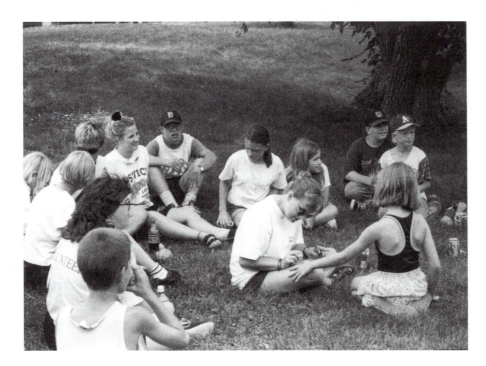

On a 5-point scale from 1 (*I never do*) to 5 (*I always do*) rate yourself on the following skills

FORMING SKILLS
(Skills needed to build initial trust in a partnership)

_____ I encourage everyone to participate
_____ I use members' names
_____ I use no "put-downs"
_____ I get to meetings on time
_____ I ask for opinions and elaboration

FUNCTIONING SKILLS
(Skills needed to manage and organize team activities so tasks are completed and relationships are maintained)

_____ I offer ideas

_____ I state and restate the purpose of the meeting

_____ I offer procedures on how to most effectively do a task

_____ I volunteer for tasks

_____ I express support and acceptance

_____ I ask for help, clarification, or technical assistance

_____ I offer to explain or clarify

_____ I show enthusiasm and optimism

_____ I am nonjudgmental of others' contributions

FORMULATING SKILLS
(Skills needed to stimulate creative problem solving and decision making)

_____ I summarize what has been discussed

_____ I encourage assigning of specific roles

_____ I seek accuracy of information by adding to summaries or questioning

_____ I ask for feedback in a nonconfrontational way

FERMENTING SKILLS
(Skills needed to manage controversy and conflict and to stimulate refinement of solutions)

_____ I see ideas from the other person's perspective

_____ I criticize ideas without criticizing people

_____ I integrate different ideas/opinions into a single position

_____ I ask for justification of others' conclusions or ideas

_____ I extend or build on others' ideas

_____ I help to decide next steps

_____ I generate additional strategies

_____ I test reality of ideas by assessing the feasibility of their implementation

_____ I help to compromise, to harmonize

Chapter 7

What Are Challenges to Inclusion?

According to experts in the field, as well as national survey results, people with disabilities are continuously being denied access in programs and services due to a number of barriers that exist in the community (Burkhour, 1992; Dattilo, 2002; National Organization on Disability, 2000; Schleien, Ray & Green, 1997; Americans with Disabilities Act [P.L. 101-336]). A barrier is an obstruction that prohibits movement, personal growth, and/or access to community resources (Burkhour, 1992). Barriers can be viewed as challenges to be met and overcome.

There can be physical, attitudinal, communication, and language barriers. Barriers can be external (within society or the environment) or internal (within the individual). If we want to build inclusive communities, we need to inform community recreation providers, as well as the general public, of the skills and resources needed to break down those barriers. Removing barriers for inclusive programs creates an environment that welcomes and encourages all participants regardless of ability level.

For people with disabilities, the following barriers or challenges impede participation. This list of barriers is compiled from research in the field as well as from focus groups and discussions with people with disabilities (Anderson & Heyne, 2000). These barriers must be addressed so that people with disabilities have the same opportunities for recreation that other community citizens have. If we view barriers as challenges to be met and overcome, positive change can and will happen. If we view barriers as permanent and lacking solutions, then little change will occur and people with disabilities will continue to be excluded from our recreation programs and our communities.

Two people look out the same jail bars. One sees mud, the other sees stars.
—F. Langbridge

How do you view barriers to inclusion?

Attitude

Attitude (and related behavior) is the number one challenge faced by people with disabilities. The treatment of people with disabilities over the years has perpetuated negative thoughts and behaviors (J. Johnson, personal communication, 1996).

Negative attitude (and related behavior) is the number one barrier faced by people with disabilities.

- Some people without disabilities feel that people with disabilities should be segregated from the rest of society.

- Some people without disabilities feel sympathy and pity toward people with disabilities that may result in a sense of helplessness, dependence, and/or humiliation among people with disabilities.

- Some people without disabilities tend to belittle, ridicule, or even joke about people with disabilities, which can result in people with disabilities feeling devalued by society.

- Some people without disabilities ignore or avoid people with disabilities, treating them as if they do not exist or as if their disability is contagious.

- Some people without disabilities have a patronizing attitude toward people with disabilities, talking to them and treating them like small children.

Treat people with disabilities as you would like to be treated.

The attitude and the behavior exhibited in your agency and within your staff toward people with disabilities set the tone for the level of acceptance and the success of inclusion programs. According to Dattilo (2002), the attitudes of professionals providing leisure services play a critical role in supporting equal access to their programs.

Each person is calibrated by experience, almost like a measuring instrument for difference, so discomfort is informative and offers a starting point for new understanding.
—Mary Catherine Bateson

An injustice against one human being is an injustice against humanity.
—Anne Frank

Lack of Awareness

Most recreation and leisure services providers are not aware of the needs of people with disabilities or how to plan and prepare for inclusive programs. Most of us did not grow up with people with disabilities in our communities or in our classrooms. As adults we may not understand or become afraid of people with disabilities. We may not know how to interact and communicate with them.

Because society has segregated people with disabilities, it is hard to become aware, to develop an understanding, or even to build friendships with people with disabilities. Fear of people with disabilities may affect the decisions we make in our jobs and personal lives. We may not even be aware of the how this fear affects the choices we make in regards to interacting and serving people with disabilities in our programs.

Inaccessible Facilities

The inability to enter a facility or to use a service due to physical barriers hinders the participation of people with disabilities in community recreation programs. A *physical barrier* is a condition of the physical environment that restricts or complicates access, movement, or participation by individuals as they attempt to use recreation facilities or areas (Burkhour, 1992). Some examples of physical barriers include stairs, sand, curbs, narrow hallways, high countertops, pathways, uneven terrain, and heavy doors. These barriers obstruct the physical movement of people with mobility impairments in the areas of transportation, recreation participation, communication, and employment. (Standards and guidelines available to assist in designing barrier-free environments were discussed in Chapter 3.)

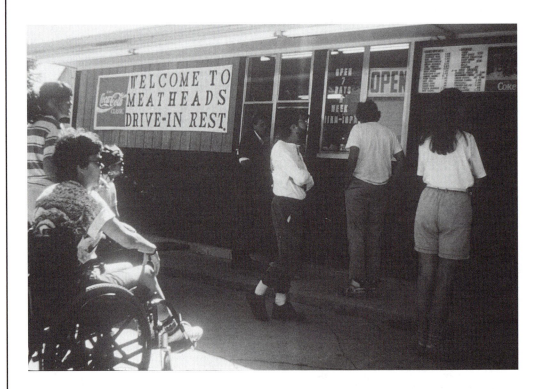

Inaccessible Programs

Segregated programs tend to be viewed as the "choice" for people with disabilities. The focus of service provision may be placed on the segregated choice at the expense of other inclusive programs.

Many community recreation programs do not have the appropriate supports needed to include persons with disabilities into regular recreational programs. Many recreational programs and activities tend to be competitive in nature. Competition tends to become exclusionary to people with less ability because it rewards only those who excel at a skill. Therefore, an array of programs, from competitive to cooperative, should be offered.

Opportunities for cooperative social interaction, self-acceptance, and fun must be nurtured, rather than ignored, in the games and sports we play. Many staff members planning and leading recreation programs have been exposed primarily to competitive activities. To provide opportunities for cooperative learning and cooperative interaction, for people with and without disabilities, one needs to foster the attitude of "cooperative programming" in all staff. If cooperative games can be used to prevent social isolation and to facilitate positive social interaction they will be of immense value to both participants with and without disabilities, including those who are shy or withdrawn and those who lack the confidence to speak up for themselves.

Inaccessibility in programs can be caused by
- Overreliance on segregated programs
- Lack of supports
- Overly competitive programming
- Lack of cooperative programming

Inadequately Trained Staff

Many recreation/leisure service agencies feel that their staff is not adequately trained to meet the individual needs of people with disabilities in their programs. Also, human service agencies may feel there is a lack of welcoming by recreation staff in their community.

Many staff members feel it is someone else's responsibility to provide recreation services to people with disabilities. Some staff feel unprepared or that they lack the skills and knowledge to work with people with disabilities.

Often recreation and leisure services providers want to include people with disabilities into their ongoing programs, they just don't know how. Proper training and education on working with people with disabilities will allow for a greater understanding and an increased comfort level for all staff.

Proper training for all agency staff on disabilities and inclusion is key to providing successful inclusive programs.

Lack of Administrative Support

For inclusion to be successful in any agency, there must be support from the agency leaders and administrators. A philosophy of providing services to everyone, regardless of ability level, needs to be shared by everyone, from the board of directors to part-time and volunteer staff. This philosophy of inclusion must emanate from a true desire to serve all people well, not "because we have to because of ADA."

A lack of support for inclusion on the part of administrators can affect the motivation of front-line staff in implementing inclusion in programs and services. Human and fiscal resources must be committed by administrators to support the inclusion efforts of the staff leading programs. Staff who work hard at and excel at providing quality recreation services to participants of all ability levels should be recognized for their efforts.

A philosophy of inclusion must be embraced enthusiastically, not grudgingly, by all agency administrators.

Role Confusion

Another challenge to recreation inclusion is confusion over who is responsible for programming services for people with disabilities. The stigma of viewing people with disabilities as helpless individuals who cannot participate in recreation programs or become full members of our communities has created a gap in the service system (Dattilo, 2002). There is a myth that people with disabilities need medical services, not community services used by "normal" people.

Many recreation and leisure service agencies have been providing segregated programs for people with disabilities. There is confusion on how to move to providing inclusive programs. Recreation and leisure service providers feel that human service agencies should be providing the programs for people with disabilities. Human service providers feel that recreation and leisure service providers should be providing the programs. Unfortunately, this lack of communication regularly results in no services being provided.

Human service providers, such as group homes, will often provide recreation services to people with disabilities within their own programs instead of using services that already exist in community recreation programs. This can lead to duplication of services or poorer quality services (e.g., grocery shopping and van rides become the primary recreation activities). Human service providers often bring large segregated groups of people with disabilities to community recreation facilities during off-hours. Not only does this deny people with disabilities the opportunity to make friends with or to recreate with people without disabilities, it also perpetuates the misperception that people with disabilities are being integrated.

Lack of Networks and Resources

Integration is a team effort and involves tapping into existing resources and working together to increase the opportunity for inclusive programs. A lack of communication often exists between professionals working in different systems. Many professionals have skills and knowledge in recreation and leisure programming, and many professionals have skills and knowledge in working with people with disabilities. Yet, if they do not know each other it is hard to communicate and to share resources and expertise. Agencies not working together to utilize each other's services may lead to a lack of inclusive recreation programs as well as a lack of support for serving people with disabilities in general. Because networking and collaboration take time and energy, many agencies have not developed strong working partnerships with other service providers. However, once networks are established and communication is strong, the returns are great for those involved. Eventually this saves time, energy, and resources.

When asking *Who should provide recreation services to people with disabilities?* one only needs to ask *Who should provide recreation services to people in general?*

Appreciation is a wonderful thing: It makes what is excellent in others belong to us as well.
—Voltaire

Assignment

Strategies To Meet Challenges and To Overcome Barriers

What challenges does your agency experience when attempting to provide inclusive recreation programs? In the following exercise a number of challenges to inclusive recreation services are listed in the left-hand column. In the right-hand column, list strategies that would assist your agency in meeting the challenge, if it exists. Do this assignment in a small group for maximum brainstorming and creativity.

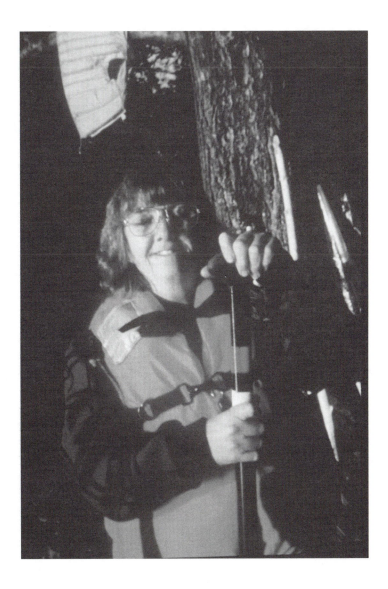

Challenge	Strategies To Meet This Challenge
Negative attitudes and related behaviors	• _____ • _____ • _____
Lack of awareness	• _____ • _____ • _____
Inaccessible facilities	• _____ • _____ • _____
Inaccessible programs	• _____ • _____ • _____
Inadequately trained staff	• _____ • _____ • _____
Lack of administrative support for inclusion	• _____ • _____ • _____
Role confusion	• _____ • _____ • _____
Lack of networks and resources	• _____ • _____ • _____

Appendix A
Rural Recreation Integration Project

The Rural Recreation Integration Project (RRIP)—a collaborative effort of the North Dakota Parks and Recreation Department and the University of North Dakota—was a 3-year project partially funded by the U.S. Department of Education, Office of Special Education and Rehabilitative Services (Award #H128J30112). It challenged itself to bridge the gap between the recreation delivery system and the human service system. It intended to develop and to sustain naturally occurring networks where resources and expertise could be shared to most effectively meet the recreation needs of people with disabilities in their communities.

The purpose of the RRIP was to facilitate the physical and social inclusion of people with disabilities into existing community recreation and leisure programs and services. The two primary activities of the RRIP were training and technical assistance. Certified therapeutic recreation specialists provided training and technical assistance to aid in the development of skills, knowledge, and networks of leisure service providers and human service providers as they worked to include people with disabilities.

Intensive training was conducted over a 3-year period to 250 people who worked in a variety of professional areas in parks and recreation and in human services. Participants in the training included people with disabilities and their family members, park directors, social workers, recreation specialists, group home managers, special education teachers, youth directors, Girl Scout staff, and advocacy groups. The training was conducted over a 2-month period each year. Because North Dakota and northwestern Minnesota are large and sparsely populated, an interactive video network was used to conduct the training (Anderson, Brown & Soli, 1996). Through a series of classrooms connected by video technology across the state, people were able to attend the training in or very near their home community. The training focused on disability awareness, physical and program accessibility, and implementation of inclusion in parks and recreation programs. During the training, participants formed partnerships composed of a human service provider and a leisure service provider. Examples of partnerships included

- Girl Scout council and an Arc chapter
- City parks and recreation district and a group home system
- State park and a disability advocacy group
- YMCA youth sports leagues and a special recreation center
- Park district summer playground program and a parent advocacy group
- Gymnastics club and a school district adaptive physical education program

Together the partners worked to include at least three people with disabilities in recreation programs. Assignments were completed during the training, but much of the work of implementing inclusion occurred after the training concluded, with technical assistance provided by the project therapeutic recreation specialists.

Technical assistance varied to meet the needs of each partnership. Examples of technical assistance included

- Staff training on disability awareness and inclusion to YMCA summer camp staff
- Assistance to a parent advocacy group to plan, implement, and evaluate a friendship/inclusion program
- Review and revision of a park district's spring/summer schedule and registration form to be more inclusive
- Disability awareness training to a church youth group
- Provision of leisure education to people living in group homes, with a focus on how to access community recreation resources
- Training for peer advocates in a gymnastics program to facilitate inclusion of children with disabilities
- Assistance with the development of before-school and after-school programs inclusive of all children
- Assistance with development of a position for an inclusion specialist to be shared by four recreation agencies
- Accessibility survey and transition plan for a Girl Scout camp

In addition, technical assistance included the development and use of an adaptive recreation equipment loan library, provision of staff training, needs assessments, and other supports for agencies. Project staff worked from an agency level to an individual level, helping children and adults with disabilities and their families to be included in the recreation activities of their choice in their communities.

Through the RRIP, we raised awareness and improved skills of recreation and human service providers, allowing them to better serve people with disabilities in their own communities. The participants who completed the formal training with the project showed a significant increase in positive attitudes toward people with disabilities and in their knowledge of inclusion strategies. The majority of the training participants implemented inclusion at their agencies, working in partnerships to better utilize expertise and resources. Mary Jo's story (p. 75) is just one example of the impact the project had on individuals' lives. System change occurred as well, with agencies changing their mission, policies, and procedures to be more inclusive. Some communities formed advisory committees to work on community issues in the area of recreation. Partnerships were formed between people with disabilities, recreation service providers, and human service providers. The RRIP can be though of as a pebble thrown in the water, with ripples spreading across the state and region. The project raised awareness and increased opportunity for people with disabilities to be a part of inclusive recreation services.

The Rural Recreation Integration Project would not have been possible without the tremendous support of the North Dakota Parks and Recreation Department. The Department fully supported the accomplishments and endeavors of the project, providing state-level leadership needed in a project of this scope. The RRIP was also supported by the following: The North Dakota Recreation and Parks Association, the Bremer Foundation, and the North Dakota Association for the Disabled. The project director was Lynn Anderson, CTRS, and the project coordinators were Carla Brown Kress, CTRS and Patricia Soli, CTRS.

> *We believe that integration and inclusion will become buzz words of years past as we move into the future where all people participate equally and share the same quality of life experiences.*

—North Dakota Parks and Recreation Department

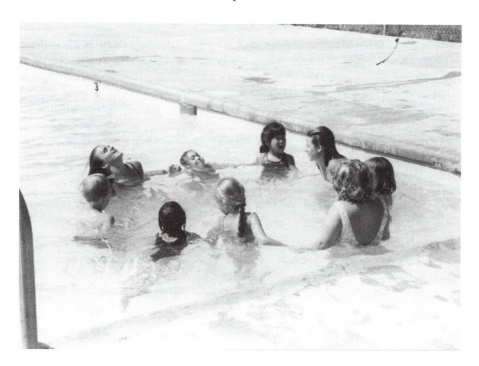

The Doors Are Opening: Mary Jo's Story
by Virginia Esslinger, Mother

As I drove up to the school door, Mary Jo said, "I go by myself; you stay here!" I inquired, "Do you remember where the meeting room is?" She replied with an emphatic "Yes!" So I remained in the car as my vivacious, dark-haired, 11-year-old daughter, who happens to have Down syndrome, bounded out of the car and closed the door. As she was getting out of the car, three of her fellow Girl Scout troop members were getting out of their cars and coming toward the school door. I heard, "Hi, Mary Jo," and "I like your new glasses." I watched as they all walked together and headed for the Junior Girl Scout meeting.

Every parent wants his or her child to be involved and socially accepted. Those of us who parent children with disabilities want this for our children as much, if not more, than parents of children without disabilities. Sometimes, for our children, it doesn't come easily. When Mary Jo first joined a Brownie troop, she was fortunate to have a troop leader who was very matter-of-fact and accepting of the fact that Mary Jo had Down syndrome. Mary Jo truly loved being a part of the Brownie troop, so when she was too old for Brownies, she "flew up" to Junior Girl Scouts. There was not a troop at her grade level in her school (where she is fully included in a regular classroom) so she was assigned to a troop in a neighboring school. The leaders were accepting of her; however, at times they seemed a bit tentative about dealing with her. Then one evening, a member of the Rural Recreation Integration Project (RRIP) spoke to the Girl Scout leaders. The next day, one of the leaders of Mary Jo's troop told me about what they had learned and how helpful the information provided had been to them. Both leaders now actively find ways to make sure that Mary Jo is fully included in all activities of the troop and seem much more comfortable with her. This is important, as the girls in the troop will take their cue from the leaders. If the leaders model acceptance and ways of including Mary Jo, the girls will learn from them and act accordingly.

The girls seem to accept Mary Jo as a member of the troop. They always greet her, include her in games and activities, and assist her when she needs (and will accept) help. Mary Jo truly enjoys being a part of the Girl Scout troop. She always remembers the meetings and is excited about going. She is learning to interact socially with children outside of her own school, the discipline provided in the Girl Scout program, and all kinds of other things from speakers and activities.

One evening last year, we received a call from Mary Jo's gym teacher at her school. The teacher said that they were just finishing a unit on gymnastics and she noticed that Mary Jo had really enjoyed it and seemed to do quite well, given her gross motor delays. She suggested that we consider enrolling her in a gymnastics club to continue with gymnastics. She met us at the gymnastics club and introduced us to the coordinator. They explained that they had both been taking classes provided by the RRIP and were looking for children with disabilities to enroll in gymnastics. Mary Jo has been involved in gymnastics ever since. She has made gains in motor ability, balance, coordination, and self-discipline, and has met many other girls from around the city. We believe her gymnastics experience contributed to her ability to finally learn to ride her bike without training wheels. The most important factor is that she truly enjoys gymnastics. She looks forward to going and participates fully with the other children in her classes. Had it not been for her gym teacher participating in the RRIP, Mary Jo may have missed this wonderful opportunity.

There is no question in our minds that the RRIP has had a positive impact on Mary Jo's life. Although she has Down syndrome, she has goals and dreams just like other children. Her goals include living as independently as possible in this community, and doing all the things that other people do, like working, having friends, and having fun. The relationships she is forming and the relationship skills she is learning through recreational activities are very precious and important to her and to us. We know we will not always be around to advocate for her. Her friends and community will have to help with that by having inclusion as an integral part of life. The RRIP has enhanced that process. The doors are opening and Mary Jo wants to go through them with her friends.

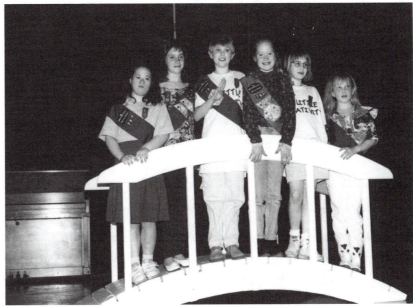

Reprinted with permission from TASH Newsletter (April 1998) and Virginia Esslinger

Appendix B
What Do I Need To Know About Disabilities To Provide Inclusive Recreation Services?

Disability is much more prevalent than many people think. The following information is taken from research conducted by the National Organization on Disability (2000a, 2000b) and from research conducted by the U.S. House of Representatives in 1990, as the Americans With Disabilities Act was being written.

- There are approximately 49,000,000 Americans with one or more physical or mental disabilities (1 in 5), and this number is increasing as the population as a whole is growing older.

- Historically society tended to isolate and segregate individuals with disabilities, and despite some improvements, some forms of discrimination against individuals with disabilities continue to be serious and pervasive problems.

- Discrimination against individuals with disabilities persists in employment, public accommodations, education, housing, transportation, communication, recreation, health services, institutionalization, voting, and access to public services.

- Individuals with disabilities continually encounter various forms of discrimination, including intentional exclusion and the discriminatory effects of architectural, transportation and communication barriers; overprotective rules and policies; failure to make modifications to existing facilities and practices; exclusionary qualification standards and criteria; segregation; and relegation to lesser services, programs, activities, benefits, and jobs.

- People with disabilities are less satisfied with their lives than people without disabilities and are much less likely to participate in their communities and to socialize.

- The nation's goals regarding individuals with disabilities are to ensure equality, opportunity, full participation, independent living, and economic self-sufficiency for such individuals.

Types of Disabilities

When working with people with disabilities, remember that the disability is just a part of the person. Also, each person who has a disability has their own individual needs. The descriptions that follow are only guidelines for you to keep in mind when working with people with various disabilities. These descriptions and suggestions are very broad and each person who has that type of disability does not necessarily possess every characteristic of the disability. Remember, ask the person with the disability what he or she needs to participate in the recreation program—don't assume anything based on type of disability.

The following provides you with information on types of disabilities, as well as some suggestions to use when working with people with disabilities. Three resources were particularly helpful in developing these suggestions:

1. National Information Center for Children and Youth with Disabilities (NICHCY, 2000) *Fact Sheets*

2. *Training Manual for ADA Compliance in Parks and Recreation Settings* by Dr. Carol Stensrud (1993)

3. *Project LIFE* materials produced by the Center for Recreation and Disability Studies (Bullock, McCann & Palmer, 1994)

Developmental Disabilities

The federal definition of a developmental disability is a severe, chronic disability of a person age 5 or older that

- Is attributable to a mental or physical impairment or combination of mental or physical impairments

- Is manifested before the age of 22

- Is likely to continue indefinitely

- Results in substantial limitations in three or more of the following areas of major life activities: self-care, receptive and expressive language, learning, mobility, self-direction, capacity for independent living, and economic self-sufficiency

Common types of developmental disabilities include attention deficit disorder, autism, cerebral palsy, mental retardation, Down syndrome, and learning disability.

Attention Deficit/Hyperactivity Disorder

Attention deficit/hyperactivity disorder (ADHD) is an impairment that interferes with the ability of the child to attend to an activity long enough to accomplish the task. ADHD is a developmental disorder of attention span, impulsivity, and/or overactivity, and rule-governed behavior (e.g., commands, directions, and instructions).

- Some people with ADHD have excessive movements that appear to be beyond their control. They have trouble sitting still and tend to fidget frequently.

- Some people with ADHD are easily distracted, have short attention spans, and are unable to concentrate. They are unable to focus or follow directions in environments that have too much stimulation, either visual or auditory.

- Some people with ADHD overreact or underreact to situations without thinking through the consequences. They tend to talk constantly and have trouble comprehending what is being said.

Suggestions When Working With People With ADHD

- Get the person's attention before talking to them.
- Keep instructions simple.
- Keep directed activity periods short.
- Arrange for the participant to sit near the leader during group activity times, when attending or participating becomes a problem.
- Limits, rules, and consequences should be clearly stated and carried out consistently.
- Maintain daily routines as much as possible.
- Try to create situations in which the participant can interact positively with peers and not become overstimulated or frustrated.
- Try to determine which activities seem to calm the child and which circumstances seem to overstimulate.
- Try to create an environment with space for active movement that can be used often throughout the day but also has enclosed areas in which the participant will be less easily distracted.
- For children, use corners of rooms for different types of learning activities, including a quiet area that can be used for nonpunitive "calming down" or "cool-off" space, with some blocks or other recreation supplies.

Autism

Autism is a complex developmental disability that typically appears during the first 3 years of life. Autism impacts the normal development of the brain in areas of

- Social interaction skills (difficulty relating to others and the outside world)
- Communication skills (both verbal and nonverbal)
- Leisure and play skills
- Uneven intellectual development (may be a genius in one area, but unable to completed daily tasks)
- Rituals and compulsiveness
- Resistance to change

Suggestions When Working With People With Autism

- Transitioning from activity to activity may be difficult. Allow for a tour of the facility in which the program takes place. Allow the participant to sit and watch the activity before participating. Sing songs from one activity to the next or have the participant carry some supplies to the next activity. This will allow the participant to develop a level of comfort before and during the program.
- Provide a picture book that includes pictures of the activities that take place during the program (e.g., sports, playground, free time, snacks, bathroom break). This will allow the participant to be prepared as to what to expect and hopefully make the transition much smoother.
- Talk with the parent or guardian to find out what motivates the participant. Include those reinforcers in your program plan.
- Allow for choice. Provide a number of activities at one time. Put children in small groups and have them rotate around to each activity. Ring a bell when it is time to change activities—they will then know time is up.
- Know the activities you are leading well. Have the parent/guardian share the participant's safety skills with you. Implement a plan to assist in teaching other needed safety skills to the participant.

Cerebral Palsy

Cerebral palsy is a condition caused by injury to parts of the brain that control our ability to use our muscles and bodies. *Cerebral* means having to do with the brain. *Palsy* means weakness or problems using the muscles. People with cerebral palsy may have difficulty controlling voluntary muscle movement.

This condition is usually caused by a lack of oxygen to the brain, resulting in permanent brain damage. The damage usually occurs during pregnancy, immediately before birth, or during birth. There are also other causes of brain damage, such as car accidents, that result in conditions resembling cerebral palsy. Not all the symptoms may show until the child is about 18 months of age, after which time this condition is nonprogressive. At times there may also be problems in speech, swallowing, vision, hearing, and/or perception.

There are various types of cerebral palsy. People who have cerebral palsy may experience loss of coordination of the muscles, difficulty with rapid or fine motor movements, spastic movement, or floppy movements of the fingers, toes, hands, and feet. Gross motor skills and mobility may be affected. A person with cerebral palsy may have hemiplegia (paralysis on one side of the body—e.g., the left arm and left leg), paraplegia (paralysis of the lower extremities), or quadriplegia (paralysis of all four quadrants of the body).

Suggestions When Working With People With Cerebral Palsy

- Allow for physical adaptations, as some people with cerebral palsy will use assistive devices like wheelchairs, walkers, and/or braces. Be prepared to make adaptations.
- Allow for communication adaptations such as TDD/TTY. Verbal language for people with cerebral palsy may be difficult to understand. Some people with cerebral palsy may use a communication board or computer. For those with no communication device, have them write down or show you what they are trying to say. Be patient.
- If you do not understand a person's speech pattern, restate what you thought was said and request clarification for what you did not understand. It is better to show the person you really want to understand rather than to pretend to understand.
- Grasping large and small objects may be difficult. Add foam handles for better grasping and allow for hand-over-hand assistance as needed for the activity (e.g., batting, coloring)
- Peer advocates work well, as they understand the disability better and are always willing to kick a ball for the participant, while another peer pushes them to first base.
- If the participant uses a wheelchair, be sure to be familiar with appropriate transfer techniques as well as the use and care of wheelchairs.
- Do not assume that the participant with cerebral palsy wants assistance, even if it looks like they are struggling with something. Ask if you can help before jumping in with assistance.

Mental Retardation

Mental retardation refers to substantial limitations in present functioning. Mental retardation manifests before age 18 and is characterized by significantly subaverage intellectual functioning, existing concurrently with related limitations in two or more of the following adaptive skill areas: communication, self-direction, health, self-care, home living, safety, social skills, functional academics, community use, leisure, or work.

Down Syndrome

There are many specific types of mental retardation. The most common and readily identifiable chromosomal condition associated with mental retardation is Down syndrome. For some unexplained reason, an accident in cell development results in 47 chromosomes instead of the usual 46. This extra chromosome changes the orderly development of the body and brain and results in mental retardation.

If working with a person with Down syndrome, a physician's permission must be obtained for him or her to participate in activities that may flex the neck because of *atlantoaxial subluxation* (see p. 80). Activities may include swimming, gymnastics, or other activities that may require head twisting type movements. This form should be given to the parents to be signed by their doctor and kept in file for further reference (NICHCY, 2000).

Suggestions When Working With People With Mental Retardation

- Use concrete, interesting, age-appropriate, and relevant materials. Because they function at a lower intellectual level does not mean you should provide activities that meet their IQ level. Instead, focus on the participant's age, and provide activities that same-age participants without disabilities would do.
- Present information and instructions in small, sequential steps and review each step frequently. Allow the participant to sit back and watch the activity before participating. Explain to them how to play the activity while the activity is going on. Listening to instructions and watching their peers (role models) will allow them to learn how to play the activity.
- Provide prompt and consistent feedback. Let them know when they did a good job by telling them specifically what they did. For example, "Good job, Jesse. I like how you sat and listened to the story."
- Treat the participant as you would anyone else. Use the same discipline techniques that you would use for participants without disabilities. Do not treat them differently because they have a disability.
- People with mental retardation will perform as you perform. Therefore, role model your expectations, such as appropriate social skills and listening skills. Let the participant know what is expected of them and the consequences if they do not meet expectations.
- Do not treat an adult with mental retardation like a child. As the leader, role model positive and respectful interactions with the participant. You may need to correct patronizing or condescending interaction by other recreation participants in a tactful, confident manner.

Down Syndrome
Individual Medical Release for Atlantoaxial Subluxation

Participant's Name _____

Agency _____

Program Leader _____

Agency Phone Number _____

Medical research has shown that up to 15% of individuals with Down syndrome suffer from a condition known as Atlantoaxial Subluxation—a misalignment of cervical vertebrae C-1 and C-2 in the neck. This exposes individuals with Down syndrome to the possibility of injury if they participate in activities that hyperextend or radically flex the neck or upper spine.

Restriction from participation by each individual with Down syndrome in the activities listed below shall continue until he/she has been examined (including x-ray views of full extension and flexion of neck) by a physician who has been briefed on the nature of the Atlantoaxial Subluxation condition and the results of such examination demonstrate that the individual does not have the condition.

Restricted Activities			
	Dance	Gymnastics	Any warm-up exercise
	Diving	High Jump	placing undue stress
	Butterfly Strokes	Skiing/Snowboarding	on the head and neck
	Soccer	Wrestling	

Physician Statement
On examination of cervical vertebrae C-1 and C-2 full flexion and full extension, I find the above named participant to have (check one)

_____No evidence of Atlantoaxial Subluxation

_____Positive or equivocal evidence of Atlantoaxial Subluxation

_____   _____
Physician's Signature   Please Print Name of Physician

_____   _____
Date Examined   Clinic or Hospital

_____   _____
Phone Number (Physician)   Address

Adapted from Heyne, L., revised edition (1992), St. Paul Jewish Community Center, St. Paul, MN

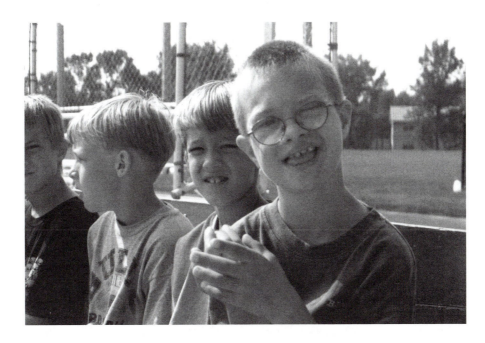

Learning Disability

A learning disability is a disorder that affects a person's ability to interpret incoming information and to link information in the brain. A learning disability is not the same as mental retardation, as most people with learning disabilities have average or above average intelligence. A learning disability can cause difficulty with spoken or written language, coordination, self-control, or attention. Learning disability is a broad term that covers many types of disability. These include developmental speech and language disorders, academic skills disorders, and coordination disorders.

Suggestions When Working With People With Learning Disabilities
• Capitalize on the participant's strengths, as the learning disability is not a pervasive disability.
• Provide structure and clear, concrete expectations. Use short sentences and simple vocabulary. Help participants to organize themselves and to manage their time during an activity.
• Allow flexibility in terms of accommodations. For example, have a written explanation of the rules of the activity in addition to the verbal explanation.
• Provide positive reinforcement. Do not embarrass the participant by asking him or her to do a task that will draw attention to the disability (e.g., writing out the group's suggestions on the chalkboard).
• If the participant has difficulty with coordination, be sure to analyze the activities for any safety issues and to manage any identified risks.

Mental Illness

Mental illness is probably the least understood and the least talked about disability. It describes a broad range of illnesses, diseases, impairments, or symptoms thought to be a result of abnormal brain function, environmental stress, or a combination of these and other factors.

- One in ten people will face a mental health problem at one point in their lives.
- About 5% of Americans have a serious mental illness.
- One in four families has a member who suffers from a mental illness.
- Only one in five people who has a mental illness seeks the help that he or she needs due to stigma, lack of awareness, or other barriers.
- About 12 million children under the age of 18 suffer from mental disorders.

The most common types of mental illness include depression, bipolar disorder, schizophrenia, and anxiety and personality disorders.

Depression

Depression is the most common form of mental illness. Symptoms include depressed mood, loss of interest or pleasure in activities, significant weight gain or loss, decrease in energy level and involvement in physical activity, and change in sleep patterns (sleeping all the time or insomnia).

Bipolar Disorder

Bipolar disorder is also called manic depression. During the manic phase, individuals have intense mood swings, exhibit endless energy, need little or no sleep, laugh at inappropriate times, or have grandiose ideas. The other side of these mood swings are depressed moods (see previous section) These episodes can last for weeks or months.

Schizophrenia

Schizophrenia is a type of psychosis, which means a person may lose touch with what is real and what is not. A person may have difficulty with unclear, confusing thoughts; may have hallucinations; or may have very low self-esteem, high anxiety, and difficulty interacting with others.

Anxiety and Personality Disorders

Individuals with these disorders suffer from many emotional conflicts in fulfilling their needs. They have difficulty dealing with their emotions and constantly feel anxious or tense. Some types of anxiety and personality disorders include phobias, panic attacks, obsessive–compulsive disorder, and hysteria.

Suggestions When Working With People With Mental Illness

The following suggestions, although broad generalizations, may be helpful to you when interacting and/or working with a person with a mental illness for the first time.

- Some people with mental illness may have difficulty with concentration due to loss of motivation, depression, and drowsiness caused by medications. Slow down. Give simple, direct instructions with an activity.
- Various medications used to treat mental illness may cause side effects such as tremors, slurred speech, excessive thirst, and extreme sensitivity to the sun. These side effects can be very frustrating to a person with a mental illness—give the person extra time or accommodations as needed. Be careful in the sun, provide water and restroom breaks, and avoid serving caffeinated beverages.
- Keep in mind that a person with mental illness may have difficulty with concentration or anxiety, which may interfere with learning. This is not due to cognitive deficits or mental retardation. Keep adult level interaction appropriate.
- Really get to know the individual and focus on their strengths. The more you know about the participant, the better able you are to help them to be included. Find out from them what works and doesn't work to help them in social situations.
- Create an atmosphere that celebrates diversity. Everyone in the group does not have to act or be the same. Create a group norm that is more accepting of a wider range of behaviors that are not disruptive or harmful. If a participant's behavior is inappropriate, let them know of a quiet place they can temporarily use to regain control. When a participant is doing well at an activity, draw attention to their participation.
- Always challenge any damaging or disparaging comments or remarks by others about mental illness. Be a constant advocate in your recreation programs. People with mental illness, no matter how serious the illness, are people first.

Physical Disabilities

A physical disability is any condition that limits a person's ability to walk, move, or interact physically with the environment. Some common functional impairments as a result of a physical disability include the following:

- Decreased muscular strength
- Limited manual dexterity and inability to grasp objects
- Lack of stamina
- Poor balance or coordination
- Poor agility
- Inability to correctly sense heat or cold

Some common types of physical disabilities include cerebral palsy, muscular dystrophy, spina bifida, spinal cord injury, head injuries (also a cognitive disability), and multiple sclerosis. Other physical disabilities that are less visible or "unseen disabilities" include asthma, heart disease, arthritis, diabetes, and pulmonary disorders. Many people with physical disabilities cannot climb stairs, walk long distances, open heavy doors, or turn doorknobs or faucet handles.

Suggestions When Working With People With Physical Disabilities

- People with physical disabilities will feel most welcome at your facility or program if the staff of your agency is familiar with some basic rules of conduct.
- Do not push a person's wheelchair or grab the arm of someone walking with difficulty. Ask first if you can be of assistance.
- Never move someone's crutches, cane, or other mobility aid without permission.
- Do not make assumptions about what a person can and cannot do. A person with a physical disability is the best judge of his or her own capabilities.
- If you offer assistance and the person declines, do not insist. If accepted, ask how you can best help.

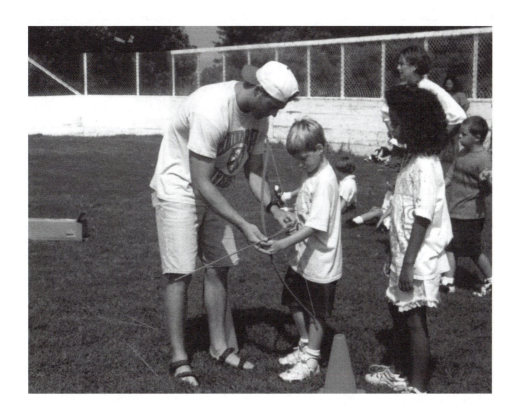

Sensory Disabilities

Hearing Impairments

Hearing impairments range from mild to profound hearing loss. People with hearing impairments include those who describe themselves as "deaf" and those who describe themselves as "hard of hearing."

Generally speaking, people who are hard of hearing have mild to severe hearing loss and often rely on amplification to assist in spoken communication. People who describe themselves as deaf generally have severe to profound hearing loss and rely heavily or entirely on visual modes of communication. People who are deaf or hard of hearing communicate with each other and with hearing people in a variety of ways, including American Sign Language (ASL), Manually Coded (Signed) English, natural gestures, reading, writing, speaking, and lip reading.

Suggestions When Working With People With Hearing Impairments

- Face the person directly and maintain eye contact. Don't turn your back or walk around while talking. If you look away, the person might assume the conversation is over. Don't cover your mouth with your hands or any object when you are speaking.
- If you are writing a message, don't talk at the same time.
- If you do not understand something that is said, ask the person to repeat it or to write it down. The goal is communication—do not pretend to understand.
- If you know sign language, try using it. It may help you to communicate and it will at least demonstrate your willingness to meet the person halfway.
- Each person should be consulted as to their type of interpreting.

Visual Impairments

People with visual impairments range from being "visually impaired" to "legally blind" to " totally blind." Within the categories of visually impaired and legally blind, wide ranges of abilities exist. Some people may be able to read large print and get around without the use of mobility aids. The disability may be more severe at night than during the day, or the extent of disability may change from day to day due to fatigue and other factors. People born with a visual impairment have a different frame of reference for spatial information, color, light, and language than people with acquired impairments who retain visual memory.

Suggestions When Working With People With Visual Impairments

- Identify yourself when you approach a person who is blind. If a new person enters, introduce them.
- Face the person and speak directly to him or her. Use a normal tone of voice.
- Don't leave without saying you are leaving.
- If you are offering assistance or directions, be as specific as possible, and point out obstacles in the path of travel, (e.g., steps, branches, curbs). For example, state, "Go five feet and turn to your left. There is a 12-inch step down after the turn."
- Never pet or otherwise distract a guide dog unless the owner has given permission.
- If a person has taken your arm, do not pull the person along. Allow the person to grip your elbow, keeping your arm relaxed.

Speech Impairments

A communication disability can result from a variety of disabilities, diseases, or disorders. Occasionally, speech impairments occur without an easily identifiable cause. An estimated two million people in the United States can hear but have difficulty with expressive communication.

Augmentative and alternative communication has developed over the years to support individuals with speech impairments. Devices range from simple communication boards on which a person points to letters, words, or pictures; to amplifiers; to sophisticated computer technology, including voice synthesizers. Not all people with speech impairments require the use of an augmentative communication device, however.

Some people who have difficulty speaking may have other physical disabilities that affect their fine and/or gross motor skills. Because it may be difficult for them to use their hands, some people with speech impairments may use a head pointer or a light stick attached to a headband to point to symbols on a communication board or to activate the computerized keyboard of their augmentative communication device. Most people who use alternative communication devices are not deaf, are not hard of hearing, and do not have a cognitive disability.

Suggestions When Working With People With Speech Impairments

When talking to people who have difficulty speaking, keep the following in mind:

- Talk to people with speech impairments as you would talk to any person.
- Be patient—it may take the person a while to answer.
- Give the person your undivided attention, as you would any person.
- Be friendly. Start up a conversation. It may be more difficult for a person with a speech impairment to get others' attention.
- Ask people with speech impairments for help in communicating with them. Often printed instructions on communication devices explain how to use them to communicate.
- Tell people with speech impairments if you do not understand what they are saying. Ask them to repeat their message, say it differently, or write it down.
- To obtain information quickly, ask short questions that require brief answers or a head nod.

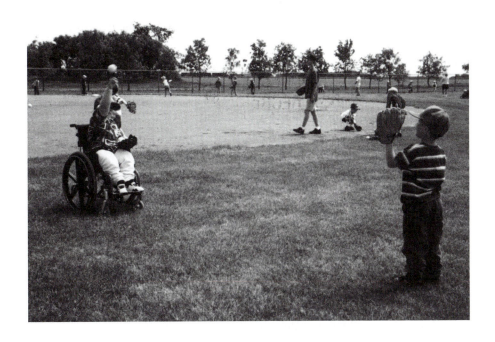

Behavior Management

Behavior describes the actions or reactions of a person under a specific circumstance. Behaviors can be seen as positive (appropriate) or negative (inappropriate). Typically in recreation programs, when behaviors occur they are negative and depend on the following:

- When   Time of behavior (e.g., always at snack time)
- Where   Situation (e.g., transitions to new activities)
- Who   Participants (e.g., another participant that seems to bring about the behavior when he or she is near the participant exhibiting the negative behavior)

Inappropriate behaviors may or may not be related to specific disabilities. Whether or not the behavior is part of the disability should not be a factor in how you deal with the situation. Each participant may exhibit inappropriate behavior throughout a program. However, dealing with the participants' behavior should be consistent across the board, regardless of ability level. The following are basic suggestions on how to deal with negative behaviors in a recreation setting:

- Be clear with other staff members as to what steps will be taken in dealing with inappropriate behavior. Everyone needs to be consistent with managing behaviors or the participants will feel empowered to act as they want and not as they are expected.

- Establish rules. Allow participants to assist in making the rules. This will allow for some ownership in acting appropriate, as the participants made the rules and will know the consequences they set for themselves. Remind the participants that rules exist to make the activity more safe and enjoyable for everyone.

- Once rules are established, make sure to follow the rules and to set a good example. Role model the type of behavior you would expect of the participants. If you are laughing and talking with other staff during story time, then the participants will think it is okay and do the same.

- Set consequences. Let the participants know the consequences when inappropriate behavior occurs.

- Follow through on your consequences. Not following through allows for increased inappropriate behavior and decreased self-control on the part of the participant, group, and program.

- Post your rules and review the rules daily before the program begins. This is a good reminder to all participants of what is acceptable and what is not.

- When inappropriate behaviors do occur, try first to redirect the participant's actions. Start a new activity or change the subject. Always try to determine what may trigger the inappropriate behavior (when, where, who) and change the circumstances in the future. Often, inappropriate behavior is another form of communication, where the participant is trying to let you know of some need not being met in the current circumstance.

- Become familiar with the conditions of the environment, such as routine, schedule, rules, and room arrangement. Get to know the participants and find out what works and what doesn't.

- Take notes as to what triggers the behavior. For example, undesired behaviors may occur during transition time, on the playground, or when sitting by another participant in particular. Also take notes on when the participant's behavior is good. Try to replicate the circumstances where appropriate behavior is most likely to occur.

- Identifying when the behavior occurs will help the participant to manage his or her behavior. For example, if transitioning from activity to activity seems difficult, have the participant carry supplies or perform some type of task to stay focused.

- Reward desired behaviors often.

- Develop a behavior plan for each program you lead. Put the behavior plan in writing. Make sure all staff, full-time and part-time, know the behavior plan and the process of administering the plan.

- Administer this policy equally with all participants, not just those who have been identified as having disabilities.

Activities to Increase Awareness of Disabilities

The following is a list of games and activities in which staff is able to simulate various types of disabilities. These are great tools for a staff training or workshop.

Interference Game

This game allows participants to simulate mental illness.

To order a copy contact
Project Life
University of Missouri
623 Clark Hall, Columbia, MO 65211
http://www.missouri.edu/~projlife/

In My Shoes

This game allows participants to simulate developmental disabilities.

To order a copy contact
The Tool Box
P.O. Box 7636, Pueblo West, CO 81007-7636
http://www.thetoolbox.org

Simulations

Appendix C provides activities to simulate various types of disabilities, including
- Attention deficit/hyperactivity disorder
- Mental retardation
- Physical disabilities
- Speech impairments
- Visual impairments
- Hearing impairments

Remember, simulations can inadvertently evoke pity for people with disabilities. A well-trained facilitator will bring about awareness of the barriers people with disabilities face without perpetuating stereotypical attitudes and pity.

The Mental Wheelchair

The wheelchair I sit in is not made of steel,
It's made of stares, and whispers, closed classroom doors, inaccessible public buildings.

And the wheelchair seems to get larger every time I'm not allowed to enter a restaurant or movie theater;
Every time people curse at me in public or try to do their "good deed."

Sitting in a wheelchair isn't bad,

It is the mental wheelchair that makes me believe I'm different, ugly,
Not touched or loved.

It's the mental wheelchair that isolates, confines, and limits me.

It's the mental wheelchair that makes me believe I'm defeated before I begin.

The wheelchair I sit in is not made of steel.

It's made of misunderstandings, ignorance, fear of the unfamiliar—of prejudice.

Why must you help it grow?

And don't you see that you, too, sit in a mental wheelchair?

So tell me, how am I different?

—Anonymous

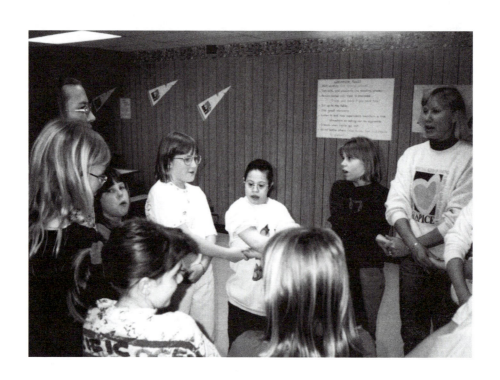

Appendix C
Simulations

Simulation Activities for
Attention Deficit/Hyperactivity Disorder (ADHD)

One at a Time

The goal of this activity is to help the participants experience the confusion of trying to follow a series of directions. Direct the participants to prepare for an activity in the usual manner without alerting them to what you plan to do. Give them 8–10 directions in your normal tone of voice, but alter the order and position of what you might expect. Example: "Please take out your math book, a pencil and sheet of notebook paper, put your name on the right side of the bottom line, the date one line up from your name on the left side and the subject two lines up from the date. Open your book to page #__ and do problems xxx, etc. Be alert to the reactions of the participants, but act as if you expect them to understand the directions.

Pinwheel Activity

Step 1: Read the instructions at a rapid pace, pausing shortly only at the designated places. Participants will experience frustration at their inability to complete the task.
Step 2: Read the instructions slowly—demonstrating each step, clarifying terms, and giving positive reinforcement as each step is completed. (Do not move to the next step until the prior step is completed.) Participants should feel successful in constructing a pinwheel with the repeat of the directions.

Directions for the Facilitator
1. Read the instructions aloud at a quick, clear pace, pausing shortly only where indicated. Participants work at completing the task according to directions given.
2. Ask participants to show what they have made and to share their feelings about the process.
3. Ask participants to explain what kinds of assistance might be given to help them feel successful about completing the task.
4. Reread instructions slowly, demonstrating, clarifying terms, giving positive reinforcement as each step is completed. (Do not move to the next step until prior step is completed.)
5. As task is completed, ask for feedback about participant's feelings and explains the relationship between this exercise and the experience of many persons with attention deficit disorder or mental retardation.

Instructions for the Activity
1. Each student is given an 8.5 x 8.5 piece of paper and tape.
2. Fold this piece of paper along the diagonal. Open it up. Fold it on the other diagonal. The diagonal means you place opposite corners on top of each other evenly and fold the paper down the middle.
3. Open up the paper. Fold it on the opposite diagonal.
4. Open up the paper. Now you have four triangles. Starting at each of the four corners of the square, cut a straight line towards the middle of the paper. Stop 1/8 inch from the center of the square.
5. This divides the square into four triangles. Now fold one of the corners of each triangle towards the center and hold it. When you have two corners in the middle, take a small piece of scotch tape and tape it down. Tape down the last two corners.
6. Now you have a pinwheel. You can take it home, find a thumbtack and a pencil with an eraser, pin the pinwheel to the eraser and you can make it spin around.

Simulation Activities for Mental Retardation

Arithmetic Exercise

Materials
Arithmetic exercise sheet, pencil

Activity
Give each participant an arithmetic exercise sheet. Give participants 3 minutes to complete the problems. If they read the directions closely, they will accomplish the activity correctly. This activity demonstrates how difficult it is for people who have mental retardation to follow complex or multistep directions.

Arithmetic Exercise

In the following simple arithmetic exercise, a "+" sign means to multiply, a "/" sign means to add, a "–" sign means to divide, and a "x" sign means to subtract. Complete the problems following these directions.

8 + 2 =	14 – 7 =	9 / 3 =
6 x 6 =	4 x 3 =	8 + 5 =
8 – 4 =	1 – 1 =	6 – 2 =
9 + 3 =	8 / 4 =	7 x 2 =
7 x 4 =	4 + 4 =	9 + 4 =
12 x 2 =	8 + 7 =	9 – 1 =
16 – 4 =	5 / 5 =	8 x 2 =
8 + 5 =	10 / 2 =	6 – 6 =

Puzzle

Materials
Puzzle pieces

Activities
Use puzzle pieces cut from large tag board. Mix pieces up and put in 4–5 envelopes (depending on number of groups). Divide the participants into 4–5 groups (depending on the size of the class) and tell them, "As a group, put the puzzle together." Allow 2 minutes and repeat directions.

You'll find each group getting frustrated because they are missing pieces—they heard you say "as a group" with the mindset of only their small group. What you want is the class as a whole group to put the puzzle together. This activity demonstrates that if explicit directions are not given to participants with mental retardation, the ability to complete a task becomes confusing and, at times, frustrating.

Simulation Activities for Physical Disabilities

Fine Motor Skills

Materials
Tape, scarves, large gloves

Activity
You are going to experience what it is like to have a fine motor disability. A fine motor disability is when the muscles in your fingers do not move easily. It is hard to do things with your hands. People who have cerebral palsy cannot move their hands very well because their brain cannot tell their hands what to do. With taped fingers, the participants attempt to perform various fine motor activities.

The participant should hold up both hands. Press fingertips together, on both hands, tape the fingertips of all 5 fingers together. The tape should be covering all the fingernails. Additionally, participants can wear gloves with taped fingers and some participants can have limited use of one arm(s) by tying one or both arms to the body.

Ideas for Activity

Object Manipulation	*Pencil/Paper Tasks*	*Self-Help Skills*	
1. scoop rice into a cup	1. print	1. button	5. buckle
2. build a tower with blocks	2. draw	2. tie	6. lace
3. string beads	3. trace	3. zip	7. eat
		4. snap	8. drink

All Thumbs

Materials
Masking tape, raisins, nuts, pudding

Activity
Sometimes people with physical disabilities don't have good muscle control. With masking tape, tape down the fingers of the person's weaker hand, leaving only the thumb free. Give each participant a cup of raisins or a dish of pudding to eat using only one hand. Divide the participants into pairs. Let one participant in each pair assist, as needed, in feeding their partner. Trade places.

Discussion
How did you feel during these exercises? Did you find ways to overcome the problems of eating when you had less control of your hands? How does it feel to be fed by someone else?

Simulation Activities for Speech Impairments

Dialogue

Materials
Marshmallows

Activity
After putting two marshmallows in their mouths, participants can either answer questions or read a statement or a question from an index card. Have each participant take turns.

Sing-a-Long

Materials
Marshmallows

Activity
All participants put a marshmallow in the middle of their mouth. Designate one leader per song to get in front of the group and lead a well-known song (e.g., Row, Row, Row Your Boat).

Simulation Activities for Visual Impairments

Blindfold (older group)

Materials
Blindfolds and paper bags with crayons, scissors, tape, and paper inside

Activity
Put on blindfolds and remind participants to keep their eyes closed under the blindfolds. Next, place a paper bag in front of each person and request that they complete the following:

- Cut a circle from the piece of paper.
- Find the crayons and tape.
- Draw a face on the circle.
- Tape the face that was drawn on the top of the large sheet of paper that was passed out.
- Draw a body under the face then write your name at the bottom of the paper.
- Clean up the work area when finished, leaving the blindfolds on.
- Put all scraps of paper in the garbage cans located at each end of the table.
- Put scissors, crayons, and tape back in the paper bag.

Instruct participants to take off their blindfolds and see how they did.

Touch and Feel Bag (younger group)

Materials
Blindfolds, bag with various objects in it

Activity
Have participants sit in a circle and put on blindfolds (if they are afraid of wearing the blindfold they can just close their eyes). Have them sit quietly for 30 seconds and listen to noises around them. Next, pass the bag around the circle and have the participants feel items and try to identify the objects.

1. Put 6 items in a bag. Name one item and have a participant find it by feeling it. Take it out for all to see. Pass the bag.

2. Put one item in a bag. Pass bag around and have each participant tell what it is by just feeling it.

3. Put very unusual items in a bag. Have one participant describe what it feels like and have the rest of the group guess what it is.

Taste Test

Materials
Related foods such as tangerines, oranges, and grapefruits

Activity
Have participants try to identify these foods by tasting and smelling only, not seeing or feeling. Have them talk about what they could tell about the foods.

Simulation Activities for Hearing Impairments

Soundless World

Materials
Short movie, written questions

Activity
Show a short, interesting movie or cartoon, such as a Disney cartoon, with the sound off. Ask the participants to write answers to some questions about the movie. Some of the questions will be about the plot that cannot be answered without hearing the script. Some should be ones that can be answered on what is seen. Show the movie again with sound. Ask the questions again. After someone answers the questions correctly, find out what some of the answers were when no one could hear them. Here are some other questions you might discuss: What were you able to understand even though you couldn't hear? What senses can a person who is deaf use to understand what's going on? What challenges would you have if you couldn't hear?

Recordings That Simulate Sounds as Heard by People With Hearing Impairments

Materials
Audiocassette of "Say What...? An Introduction to Hearing Loss," available from the American Academy of Audiology—http://www.audiology.org—simulates several types of abnormal hearing, as do links available at: http://www.neurophys.wisc.edu/animations/

Activity
As a group, listen to the audiocassette and discuss the effect a hearing impairment may have on daily life and recreation.

Appendix D
Sample Intake and Assessment Forms

On the following pages you will find samples of forms you may use or adapt to complete intake interviews or assessments at your agency.

- Intake Interview Assessment Form
- Participant Profile

Intake Interview Assessment Form

1. Describe your recreation program/service in detail to the registering participant with a disability (and/or parent/guardian, if a child).

   a. The daily and weekly schedule is…

   b. The activities are…

   c. The staffing consists of…(staff/participant ratio, role with participants, staff's background and training)

2. Ask the participant with a disability (or the parent/guardian) the following:

   a. What is your goal (for your child)? What are your expectations of the program or service?

   b. What are your (your child's) favorite activities at home, neighborhood and work/school?

   c. What are your (your child's) needs in this program or service (e.g., medical, safety, mobility, social/communication)?

   d. What do you worry about in this program? What kinds of issues may you have that we can avoid in this program?

   e. What motivates you (your child)? How do you let your child know they're doing a good job? What type of encouragement do you use (e.g., verbal praise)?

   f. Who else knows you (your child) that we can talk to (e.g., case managers, teachers, other program leaders, neighbors)? Is it OK to contact them?

3. Questions for the recreation specialist to ask the recreation staff:
   What resources within the program can we capitalize on?

   a. Setting—equipment, accessible areas?

   b. Staff—who has training and/or experience with people with disabilities?

   c. Family, friends, other participants—whom does the participant know in our program?

BLOOMINGTON, EDEN PRAIRIE, EDINA, RICHFIELD

PARTICIPANT PROFILE

Adaptive/Inclusive Recreation Learning Exchange

Date Printed: 02/12/2003

The Data Practices Act requires that we inform you of your rights about the private data we are requesting on this form. Private data is available to you, but not to the public. This information can be shared with the Recreation and Learning Exchange of the Cities and School Districts of Bloomington, Eden Prairie, Edina, Richfield, and TRAIL. You can withhold this data, but you may not receive updated program information and/or accommodations. Your signature on this form indicates you understand these rights.

Signature _____ Date _____

Last Name:	First Name:	Nickname:

Address:	City:	State:	Zip:

Birthdate:	Age:	Sex (M/F):	Home Phone:	Work Phone:

Legal Guardian (if not Self):	Relationship:	Home Phone:

Address:	City:	State:	Zip:	Work Phone:

Emergency Contact:	Home Phone:	Work Phone:

Current School Grade:	School/Work Place:	☐ Check here if it is okay to contact Teacher/Support Staff for add'l information on individual needs.
Teacher/Support Staff:	Phone:	

CHECK AS MANY AS APPLY

(Please use comments on the back of this form to explain as necessary)

COMPREHENSION

When given a one- or two-step verbal direction, the person:

☐ Always Understands	☐ Rarely Understands
☐ Usually Understands	☐ Never Understands
☐ Sometimes Understands	☐ Other

TRANSPORTATION

☐ Self	☐ Staff
☐ Parent	☐ TRAIL
☐ Guardian	☐ Other

MOST COMFORTABLE SETTING

☐ Individual	☐ Small Group
☐ Individual or Small Group	
☐ Other	

COMMUNICATION

☐ Good	☐ Dominates Conversation
☐ Shy	☐ Inappropriate Topics
☐ Limited Conversation	☐ Other
☐ Interpreter Needed	

LIVING SITUATION

☐ Independent	☐ Parent's Home
☐ Foster Home	☐ Group Home
☐ Semi-Independent	☐ Other

_____
Name of Residence or Agency

GENERAL CONCERNS

☐ Behavior
☐ Physical Limitations
☐ Allergies
☐ Other

SCHEDULING NEEDS

☐ Medication
☐ Toileting
☐ Other

DIETARY NEEDS

☐ Special Diet (see Comments on back)

RECREATIONAL GOALS

☐ Fitness	☐ Socialization
☐ Friendship	☐ Skills
☐ Other (see Comments on back)	

Profile Completed By: _____ Phone: _____

Relationship to Participant: _____ Date: _____

CHECK EACH THAT APPLIES IN ORDER TO ASSIST WITH DIRECT MAILINGS

☐ ADD / ADHD	☐ Fetal Alcohol Syndrome	☐ Mobility Impairment	☐ Speech Delay
☐ Autism / PDD	☐ Fragile X	☐ Multiple Sclerosis	☐ Spina Bifida
☐ Brain Injury	☐ Deaf / Hard of Hearing	☐ Nonverbal	☐ Tourette Syndrome
☐ Cerebral Palsy	☐ Learning Disability	☐ Nondisabled	☐ Tuberous Sclerosis
☐ Down Syndrome	☐ Mental Health	☐ Physical Disabilities	☐ Visually Impaired
☐ EBD / ODD	☐ Mental Retardation	☐ Prader-Willi	☐ Other
☐ Epilepsy	☐ Mildly Mentally Impaired	☐ Rett Syndrome	

FOR THE PARTICIPANT WITH EPILEPSY OR SEIZURES

Type of seizure(s): _____

Current medications: _____

Likelihood and frequency of seizures: _____

Stimulus or activities which may trigger a seizure: _____

Desired first-aid procedures: _____
(Our policy is to call 9-1-1 if a seizure lasts more than 3 minutes, unless otherwise requested by a parent / guardian.)

Other comments: _____

FAVORITE ACTIVITIES / OTHER

PLEASE WRITE ALL ADDITIONAL COMMENTS HERE. IF YOU NEED MORE SPACE, PLEASE CONTINUE ON ANOTHER SHEET.

Publicity: My name ☐   photograph ☐   both ☐   may be used for publicity purposes.

Return to: Adaptive Recreation Supervisor
City of Bloomington
2215 West Old Shakopee Road
Bloomington, MN 55431-3096

Appendix E
Sample Scenarios for Staff Training

Use the following scenarios to practice applying the inclusion (problem-solving) process. Keep in mind physical as well as social integration.

Scenario #1

There is a child in your recreation program who has mental retardation and also has seizures. A group of popular children ignore this child and talk about him or her to the other children. Names like "stupid," "retard," and "crazy" have been used. How do you deal with this situation?

Scenario #2

You have a child who uses a wheelchair and uses a communication board to interact with others. She wants to join her neighborhood T-ball league. What process and adaptations would you make so that she can play and participate in the game?

Scenario #3

You have an adult in your aerobics class who consistently wants to touch (e.g., hug, pat heads) the other participants and staff. This draws attention to the participant and bothers the others. How could you handle this situation?

Scenario #4

You are a program leader with a parks and recreation department. Registration is starting for this year's summer camps. A parent calls you and states: "I want to sign my child up for your 6-week day camp program. My child happens to have some significant disabilities. And by the way, I have a good lawyer." How do you handle this situation?

Scenario #5

A staff member from a psychosocial rehabilitation center for people with mental illness calls you to see if one of his clients can join the painting class your agency sponsors. How should you proceed with this situation?

Scenario #6

You have a child who uses a wheelchair and has a developmental disability. He does not speak very clearly or consistently and also drools. He enjoys your playground program and all the activities. On the first day of the program, the other kids in the group begin to ask you questions about this child: "Why does he use a wheelchair?" "Why does he drool?" "Why can't he talk right?" "Why is he at our playground?" How would you handle this situation?

Appendix F
Roles of Staff and Volunteers

Role of Program Leader in Facilitating Inclusion

A program leader can play a key role in facilitating the inclusion process. A program leader's feedback regarding the inclusion process is essential to ensure a positive integrated experience for all participants. Following are some recommendations to clarify the role a program leader plays:

- Create an atmosphere of acceptance toward the person with a disability by being a role model for the group on how to interact with the person.
- Act natural when interacting with the person with a disability. Treat the person in the same manner as you treat other participants in the program.
- When providing individual instruction, give the same amount of instruction to the person with a disability as to the other participants, whether or not the person receives a one-to-one assistant as a go-between.
- When communicating with a person with a disability, speak directly to him or her rather than use the one-to-one assistant.
- Focus on what the person *can* do, and positively reinforce those behaviors to increase their occurrence and development.
- When possible, avoid competitive activities where people can potentially be excluded from involvement. Rather, structure the activity and group to encourage cooperation to meet group goals.
- When questions arise about the participant's disability or the participant, answer to the best of your ability. Use the one-to-one assistant or ask the parent/guardian for more information.

Adapted from Heyne, L., revised edition (1992)

Role of the One-to-One Assistant (Additional Staff Person)

A one-to-one assistant is a support person for the program leader. He or she facilitates the involvement of a person with a disability in the program to the maximum degree possible. No program planning is required of the assistant except to ensure that the person with a disability can actively participate in the activity. In general, the role of the assistant includes the following responsibilities:

- Provide additional assistance (e.g., interpreting instructions, providing physical assistance) to help the participant with a disability to learn new recreation and leisure skills.
- Encourage social interaction between the participant with a disability and the nondisabled participants.
- Adapt activities as needed to allow active participation by the participant with a disability.
- Provide positive reinforcement or other behavioral intervention (as needed) to facilitate the participant's involvement in the group.
- Promote the participant's enjoyment in the program.
- Respond to any questions that arise from the nondisabled participants or the group leader regarding the person with a disability or the disability in general.

The role a one-to-one assistant plays in integrated programs requires a sensitivity as to when to offer the person with a disability individual assistance, and when to allow the natural dynamics of group interactions and instructions to assimilate the person in the group as part of a more spontaneous process. In some integrated programs, too much intervention from the assistant can inhibit socialization and learning.

Adapted from Heyne, L., revised edition (1992)

Appendix G
Sample Documentation and Evaluation Forms

On the following pages you will find samples of forms you may use or adapt to document and to evaluate inclusion at your agency.

- Goals and Progress Notes on Participant
- Integration Activity Notes
- Participant Evaluation (Child)
- Parent/Guardian Evaluation
- Participant Evaluation (Adult)
- Nondisabled Participant Evaluation
- Staff Recommendations on Participant

Goals and Progress Notes on Participant

Participant _____ Program _____

Parent/Guardian Program Goal for Child _____

Goal

Measurable Objectives (behavior, time, duration, criteria)

1.

2.

3.

Narrative Documentation

What objectives were achieved?

How were they achieved?

Recommendations/Updated Objectives

Facilitator _____

Adapted from City of Eden Prairie's Therapeutic Recreation Services Program, Eden Prairie, MN (2001)

Integration Activity Notes

Participation _____ Program _____

Documentation Week _____ Location _____

Day _____ Activity _____

Adaptations/Recommendations _____

_____

_____

Day _____ Activity _____

Adaptations/Recommendations _____

_____

_____

Day _____ Activity _____

Adaptations/Recommendations _____

_____

_____

Day _____ Activity _____

Adaptations/Recommendations _____

_____

_____

Day _____ Activity _____

Adaptations/Recommendations _____

_____

_____

Adapted from City of Eden Prairie's Therapeutic Recreation Services Program, Eden Prairie, MN (2001)

Participant Evaluation (Child)

Program _____

Yes   No

Circle the face that best describes how you feel.

1. Did you have fun?

2. Did you make new friends?

3. What did you think of the program?

4. Did you like the staff?

5. What was your favorite thing about the program?

6. What is something you didn't like about the program?

Adapted from City of Eden Prairie's Therapeutic Recreation Services Program, Eden Prairie, MN (2001)

Parent/Guardian Evaluation

Program _____   Date _____

Parent Name (optional) _____

Participant Name (optional) _____

1)   Did you feel this program was beneficial to your son/daughter?

YES _____   NO _____

Comments

2)   Do you feel the staff members created a positive experience for your son/daughter?

YES _____   NO _____

Comments

3)   Do you feel you had adequate communication between yourself and the recreation program staff and supervisor?

YES _____   NO _____

Comments

4)   If you could change anything about the program what would it be (e.g., program activities, content, organization, staff, communication)?

5)   What worked well?

6)   Suggestions for improvement

Thank you for completing this form.

Adapted from City of Eden Prairie's Therapeutic Recreation Services Program, Eden Prairie, MN (2001)

Participant Evaluation (Adult)

Program _____ Date _____

Participant Name (optional) _____

1) Did you feel this program was beneficial to you?

YES _____ NO _____

Comments

2) Do you feel the staff members created a positive experience for you?

YES _____ NO _____

Comments

3) If you could change anything about the program what would it be (e.g., program activities, content, organization, staff, communication)?

4) What worked well and what did you like about the program?

5) Suggestions for improvement or additional comments

Thank you for completing this form.

Adapted from City of Eden Prairie's Therapeutic Recreation Services Program, Eden Prairie, MN (2001)

Nondisabled Participant Evaluation

Program _____ Date _____

Participant Name (optional) _____

1) How did you feel about being in an inclusive program?

2) What did you learn regarding people with disabilities and inclusion?

3) Do you feel inclusion enhanced or hurt the group and/or program?

4) Do you have any suggestions on improving the inclusion of people with disabilities into our ongoing programs?

5) Additional comments

Thank you for completing this form.

Adapted from Heyne, L., revised edition (1992), St. Paul Jewish Community Center, St. Paul, MN

Staff Recommendations on Participant

This information is for future programs in which the participant will be involved. Use the back as needed.

Program _____ Date/Year _____

Location of Program _____

Name of Participant _____

Name of Staff Completing Form _____

1) To what extent do you feel the participant's goals were met?

2) What strategies were used to reach the goals (e.g., behavior management plan, equipment, peer advocates, one-to-one assistant)?

3) Do you feel a one-to-one assistant is needed for this participant in future programs? Explain.

4) Was the length and location of the program adequate to meet the participant's needs?

5) What would you recommend to next year's staff when working with this participant?

6) Suggestions or comments

Thank you for completing this form.

Adapted from City of Eden Prairie's Therapeutic Recreation Services Program, Eden Prairie, MN (2001)

References

Architectural Barriers Act of 1968, as amended, Pub. L. No. 90-480, 42 U.S.C. §§ 4151 et seq.

Americans With Disabilities Act of 1990, Pub. L. No. 101-336, § 2, 104 Stat. 328 (1991).

Anderson, L. (1994). *Outdoor adventure recreation and social integration: A social-psychological perspective.* Unpublished doctoral dissertation, University of Minnesota, Minneapolis, MN.

Anderson, L., Brown, C., and Soli, P. (1996). The rural recreation integration project: Reaching out with interactive video technology. *Parks & Recreation, 31*(5), 38–43.

Anderson, L. and Heyne, L. (2000). A statewide needs assessment using focus groups: Perceived challenges and goals in providing inclusive recreation service in rural communities. *Journal of Park and Recreation Administration, 18(4),* 17–37.

Berger, A. (1994). Inclusion: Not an ideology, but a way of life. *TASH Newsletter, 20*(1), 4–7.

Bullock, C., McCann, C., and Palmer, R. (1994). *LIFE resources: The LIFE resources manual.* Chapel Hill, NC: Center for Recreation and Disability Studies.

Burkhour, C. (1992). *Inclusive recreation: Planning recreation opportunities for people of all abilities.* Lansing, MI: Department of Natural Resources.

Canadian Parks/Recreation Association. (1997). *The benefits catalogue.* Gloucester, Ontario, Canada: Author.

Dattilo, J. (2002). *Inclusive leisure services: Responding to the rights of people with disabilities* (2nd ed.). State College, PA: Venture Publishing, Inc.

Esslinger, V. (1998). The doors are opening: Mary Jo's story. *TASH Newsletter, 24*(4), 27.

Goltsman, S. M., Gilbert, T. A., and Wohlford, S. D. (1993). *The accessibility checklist: An evaluation system for buildings and outdoor settings.* Berkeley, CA: MIG Communications.

Heyne, L. (1992). *Roles of staff and volunteers.* Unpublished manuscript.

Heyne, L., Schleien, S. J., and McAvoy, L. (1993). *Making friends: Using recreation activities to promote friendships between children with and without disabilities.* Minneapolis, MN: Institute on Community Integration/University of Minnesota.

Hutchison, P. and McGill, J. (1992). *Leisure, integration, and community.* Concord, Ontario, Canada: Leisurability Publications, Inc.

Jensen, L. *Language and behavior awareness survey.* Unpublished manuscript.

Johnson, D., Johnson, R., and Holubec, E. (1991). *Cooperation in the classroom.* Edina, MN: Interaction Book.

McGovern, J. (1993). *The ADA self-evaluation handbook for park districts.* Ashburn, VA: National Recreation and Park Association.

McGovern, J. (2000). *ADA.* Session presented at the Minnesota Recreation and Park Association Conference, Minneapolis, MN.

Montgomery County Department of Recreation. (1986). *Mainstreaming: A total perspective.* Silver Spring, MD: Author

National Organization on Disability. (2000a). *Harris survey of Americans with disabilities.* Retrieved from http://www.nod.org

National Organization on Disability. (2000b). *Harris survey of community participation.* Retrieved from http://www.nod.org

National Information Center for Children and Youth With Disabilities. (2000). *NICHCY fact sheets.* Retrieved from http://www.nichcy.org

Parks and Recreation Federation of Ontario. (1992). *The benefits of parks and recreation: A catalogue.* Gloucester, Ontario, Canada: Canadian Parks and Recreation Association.

Russell, R. (2002). *Pastimes: The context of contemporary leisure* (2nd ed.). Champaign, IL: Sagamore Publishing.

Rynders, J. and Schleien, S. (1991). *Together successfully: Creating recreational and educational programs that integrate people with and without disabilities.* Arlington, TX: ARC-USA.

Schleien, S. J. (1993). Access and inclusion in community leisure services. *Parks & Recreation, 28*(4), 66–72.

Schleien, S. J. and Green, F. P. (1992). Three approaches for integrating persons with disabilities into community recreation. *Journal of Park and Recreation Administration, 10*(2), 51–66.

Schleien, S. J., McAvoy, L., Lais, G., and Rynders, J. (1993). *Integrated outdoor education and adventure programs.* Champaign, IL: Sagamore Publishing.

Schleien, S. J., Ray, T., and Green, F. (1997). *Community recreation and people with disabilities: Strategies for inclusion* (2nd ed.). Baltimore, MD: Paul H. Brookes Publishing Co.

Stensrud, C. (1993). *A training manual for Americans With Disabilities Act: Compliance in parks and recreation settings*. State College, PA: Venture Publishing, Inc.

Thousand, J. and Villa, R. (1992). Interpersonal skills for effective collaboration. *Impact, 4*(3), 12–13. Minneapolis, MN: Institute on Community Integration, Univeristy of Minnesota.

Wagner, G. Wetherald, L., and Wilson, B. (1994). A model for making county and municipal recreation department programs inclusive. (pp. 181–192). In S. Moon, *Making school and community recreation fun for everyone.* Baltimore, MD: Paul H. Brookes Publishing Co.

Random House Webster's College Dictionary. (1991). New York, NY: Random House.

Additional Readings

Anderson, L., Brown, C., and Soli, P. (1998). Recreation–human service partnerships: The rural recreation integration project. *TASH Newsletter, 24*(4), 25–26.

Bullock, C. and Mahon, M. (2000). *Introduction to recreation services for people with disabilities: A person-centered approach* (2nd ed.). Champaign, IL: Sagamore Publishing.

Cangemi, P., Williams, W., and Gaskell, P. (1992). Going to the source for accessibility assessment. *Parks & Recreation, 27*(10), 66–69.

Casciotti, E. (1993). *ADA resource guide for parks, recreation and leisure service agencies.* Ashburn, VA: National Recreation and Park Association.

Clinton, H. R. (1996). *It takes a village and other lessons children teach us.* New York, NY: Simon & Schuster.

Hackett, L. K. (1994). *Everybody belongs: Tips for including your child in community recreation.* NH: Developmental Disabilities Council.

Kimeldorf, M. (1989). *Pathways to leisure.* Bloomington, IL: Meridian Education Corporation.

McAvoy, L. (1991/1992). Administrative issues in integrated outdoor programs. *Impact, 4*(4), 16. Minneapolis, MN: Institute on Community Integration, University of Minnesota.

McFadden, D. L. and Burke, E. P. (1992/1993, Winter). The ADA: What does it mean for people with developmental disabilities? *Impact, 5*(4), 1–18. Minneapolis, MN: Institute on Community Integration, University of Minnesota.

McLean, D. (1993). Partnering: Extending resources and building networks. *Parks & Recreation, 28*(12), 48–51.

Neu, S. (1991). *Partnering.* Presentation handout from the North Dakota Recreation & Parks Association Annual Conference (Steve Neu 701–222–6455).

Pearson, L., Kempf, B., Hansing, J., Blomgren, C., Brooker, G., and Fahnestock, M. (1992-93). Customer service: One city's vision of inclusion. *Impact, 5*(4), 10–11. Minneapolis, MN: Institute on Community Integration, University of Minnesota.

Schattman, R. (1991). Step by step: A system's evolution toward inclusion. *Impact, 4*(3), 6–7. Minneapolis, MN: Institute on Community Integration, University of Minnesota.

Schleien, S., Rynders, J., Heyne, L., and Tabourne, C. (1995). *Powerful partnerships: Parents and professionals building inclusive recreation programs together.* Minneapolis, MN: Institute on Community Integration, University of Minnesota.

Sykes, D. J. (1991). Staff training for inclusion. *Impact, 4*(2), 9. Institute on Community Integration, University of Minnesota.

Online Resources

Adaptive Equipment and Resources

Webpage accessibility for people with vision impairments is accomplished through design and text boxes. These websites help to design and assess accessibility for webpages.
http://www.cast.org/bobby
http://www.makoa.org/web-design.htm

Access Outdoors provides information related to accessible outdoor recreation.
http://www.accessoutdoors.org

Assistivetech.net is an online resource providing information on assistive technology, adaptive environments, community resources, and excellent recreation-related links.
http://www.assistivetech.net

Abledata is a government-funded website maintained by the National Institute on Disability and Rehabilitation Research and the U.S. Department of Education. It contains detailed descriptions and pictures of over 27,000 adaptive equipment products and companies in an easy to use searchable database. It has links to numerous recreation adaptive equipment sites and adaptive recreation programs.
http://www.abledata.com

Disability and Advocacy

American Association of People With Disabilities
http://www.aapd-dc.org

Consortium of Developmental Disabilities Councils
http://www.cddc.com

The Arc
http://www.thearc.org

Disability Films has numerous films on disability awareness that may be useful for staff training.
http://www.disabilityfilms.co.uk

Disability Resources on the Internet
http://www.disabilityresources.org

International Association of Psychosocial Rehabilitation Services
http://www.iapsrs.org

International Center for Disability Resources on the Internet
This site collects and presents many disability-related Internet resources. It has links for sport, travel, and leisure.
http://www.icdri.org

Job Accommodations Network
Advice on accommodating employees with disabilities
http://www.jan.wvu.edu

National Arts and Disability Center
An information, training, and resource center whose mission is to promote the full inclusion of people with disabilities in the visual, performing, media, and literary arts.
http://www.nadc.ucla.edu

The National Center on Accessibility (NCA), affiliated with Indiana University, provides a wealth of resources on access in parks, recreation, and tourism. The NCA website has information on training, education, research results, and newsletters, as well as links to obtain technical assistance. It has the most current updates on accessibility guidelines in recreation and outdoor recreation areas.
http://www.ncaonline.org

The National Center on Physical Activity and Disability has fact sheets on various disabilities; resource directories of organizations and programs that provide accessible physical activity, sport, and recreation; adaptive equipment vendors; bibliographies of research related to disability and activity; and adaptations for various activities.
http://www.ncpad.org

National Council on Disability
http://www.ncd.gov

National Council on Independent Living
http://www.ncil.org

The National Information Center for Children and Youth with Disabilities is a national information and referral center that provides information on disabilities and disability-related issues for families and professionals. The website contains fact sheets about specific disabilities, FAQ pages on breaking or recent news and developments in the area of disability, training materials, and a wealth of links.
http://www.nichcy.org

National Organization on Disability
http://www.nod.org

PACER Center (Parent Advocacy Coalition for Educational Rights)
612–827–2966
http://www.pacer.org

Person-centered resources and practices to support people with disabilities
http://www.qualitymall.org

TASH
http://www.tash.org

The United Way is at the forefront in building effective partnerships to meet community needs. The United Way website has a wealth of information, as well as links to local United Way chapters.
http://www.unitedway.org

Government

U.S. Access Board
http://www.access-board.gov

The following guidelines and survey forms are available on the U.S. Access Board website:
- ADA Accessibility Guidelines and Checklist (ADAAG)
- USAF Standards and Checklist

- Play Area Guidelines
- Recreation Facilities Guidelines
- Outdoor Developed Area Guidelines

U.S. Census Bureau
http://www.census.gov

U.S. Department of Agriculture
http://www.usda.gov

U.S. Department of Education
http://www.ed.gov

U.S. Department of Health and Human Services
http://www.hhs.gov

U.S. Department of Housing and Urban Development
http://www.hud.gov

U.S. Department of Interior (National Park Service, Bureau of Indian Affairs, Bureau of Land Management, U.S. Fish and Wildlife Service)
http://www.doi.gov

U.S. Department of Justice
Up-to-date information and resources about the ADA
http://www.usdoj.gov

U.S. Equal Opportunity Commission
http://www.eeoc.gov

U.S. Department of Labor, Office of Disability Employment Policy
http://www.dol.gov/odep

U.S. Department of Transportation, Office of the General Counsel for Regulation and Enforcement
http://www.dot.gov/ost/ogc/org/regulation

Federal Communications Commission, Disability Rights Office
http://www.fcc.gov/cgb/dro

The Catalog of Federal Domestic Assistance provides links to federal grant programs by topical area.
http://www.cfda.gov

For a one-stop online access to resources, services, and information about disability available throughout the federal government, use this website:
http://www.disability.gov

This site features federal land management agencies working to make outdoor recreation opportunities available to all.
http://www.recreation.gov/access.cfm

Grants

The Arc website provides official position statements for the Arc—useful for program proposal writing.
http://www.thearc.org

The Children with Disabilities website provides links to federal, state, and nonprofit foundations that provide grant opportunities in the area of disability.
http://www.childrenwithdisabilities.ncjrs.org

The Foundation Center provides searchable databases to find foundations that fund in your area of need. Also, it provides numerous listings of educational opportunities to learn more about grant writing.
http://www.fdncenter.org

Fundsnet services, although a commercial website, provides numerous links to funding agencies and foundations.
http://www.fundsnetservices.com

The Institution on Community Integration at the University of Minnesota offers several resources for grant writers seeking funding for disability-related projects.
http://www.ici.umn.edu

Independent Living Centers

The Design Linc: Accessibility Design and Resources
http://www.designlinc.com

Independent Living Research Utilization
Directory of U.S. and Canadian independent living centers
http://www.bcm.tmc.edu/ilru

National Council of Independent Living Centers
http://www.ncil.org

Leisure Interest Assessment Tools

The Leisure Diagnostic Battery
Available from Venture Publishing, Inc.
814–234–4561
http://www.venturepublish.com

The Leisure Interest Measurement
The Leisure Scope Plus
The Teen Leisure Scope Plus
The Leisure Battery
Assessment Tools for Recreational Therapy, 2nd Edition
Available from Idyll Arbor Publishing
201–432–3231
http://www.idyllarbor.com

Leisure Interest Survey
Available from CompuTR
http://www.recreationtherapy.com/computr.htm

Professional Associations

The following branches of the National Recreation and Park Association provide useful publications and educational opportunities to assist agencies in meeting administrative concerns with inclusion. All of these organizations have websites linked from the NRPA homepage.

- American Park and Recreation Society
- Armed Forces Recreation Society
- Citizen Board Member Branch
- National Society for Park Resources
- National Therapeutic Recreation Society
- Society for Park and Recreation Educators

National Recreation and Parks Association
http://www.nrpa.org

National Council for Therapeutic Recreation Certification
http://www.nctrc.org

American Therapeutic Recreation Association
http://www.atra-tr.org

Canadian Parks and Recreation Association
http://www.cpra.ca

Publications

The Institute on Community Integration (ICI) publishes *Impact*, a free quarterly newsletter and an excellent staff training resource. The ICI conducts extensive research on inclusion, provides technical assistance, and publishes an array of reports available to the public.
Institute on Community Integration
University of Minnesota
102 Pattee Hall, 150 Pillsbury Drive SE
Minneapolis, MN 55455
612–624–6300
http://www.ici.umn.edu

NRPA Law Review
This is a regular column in *Parks and Recreation Magazine*, the monthly publication of the National Recreation and Park Association (NRPA). Written by James Kozlowski (JD, PhD) it provides excellent reviews of cases that directly pertain to liability, ADA compliance, discrimination, and other relevant issues that affect administrators in parks and recreation. You can join NRPA and receive *Parks and Recreation Magazine* by visiting their website:
http://www.nrpa.org

Specific Disabilities

Attention Deficit/Hyperactivity Disorder
Attention Deficit Disorder Association
http://www.add.org

Autism
Autism Society of America
http://www.autism-society.org

Cerebral Palsy
United Cerebral Palsy
http://www.ucpa.org

Developmental Disabilities
TASH
http://www.tash.org
The Arc
http://www.thearc.org
National Down Syndrome Society
http://www.ndss.org

Hearing Impairments
National Association of the Deaf
http://www.nad.org

Learning Disabilities
Coordinated Campaign for Learning Disabilities
http://www.ldonline.org

Mental Illness
National Alliance for the Mentally Ill
http://www.nami.org

Mental Retardation
American Association on Mental Retardation
http://www.aamr.org

Physical Disabilities
Easter Seals
http://www.easter-seals.org

Speech Impairments
American Speech–Language–Hearing Association
http://www.asha.org

Spinal Injuries
National Spinal Cord Injury Association
http://www.spinalcord.org

Vision Impairments
American Foundation for the Blind
http://www.afb.org
National Federation of the Blind
http://www.nfb.org

Books by Venture Publishing

Leisure Education III: More Goal-Oriented Activities
by Norma J. Stumbo

Leisure Education IV: Activities for Individuals with Substance Addictions
by Norma J. Stumbo

Leisure Education Program Planning: A Systematic Approach, Second Edition
by John Dattilo

Leisure Education Specific Programs
by John Dattilo

Leisure in Your Life: An Exploration, Sixth Edition
by Geoffrey Godbey

Leisure Services in Canada: An Introduction, Second Edition
by Mark S. Searle and Russell E. Brayley

Leisure Studies: Prospects for the Twenty-First Century
edited by Edgar L. Jackson and Thomas L. Burton

The Lifestory Re-Play Circle: A Manual of Activities and Techniques
by Rosilyn Wilder

Models of Change in Municipal Parks and Recreation: A Book of Innovative Case Studies
edited by Mark E. Havitz

More Than a Game: A New Focus on Senior Activity Services
by Brenda Corbett

Nature and the Human Spirit: Toward an Expanded Land Management Ethic
edited by B. L. Driver, Daniel Dustin, Tony Baltic, Gary Elsner, and George Peterson

The Organizational Basis of Leisure Participation: A Motivational Exploration
by Robert A. Stebbins

Outdoor Recreation Management: Theory and Application, Third Edition
by Alan Jubenville and Ben Twight

Planning Parks for People, Second Edition
by John Hultsman, Richard L. Cottrell, and Wendy Z. Hultsman

The Process of Recreation Programming Theory and Technique, Third Edition
by Patricia Farrell and Herberta M. Lundegren

Programming for Parks, Recreation, and Leisure Services: A Servant Leadership Approach
by Donald G. DeGraaf, Debra J. Jordan, and Kathy H. DeGraaf

Protocols for Recreation Therapy Programs
edited by Jill Kelland, along with the Recreation Therapy Staff at Alberta Hospital Edmonton

Quality Management: Applications for Therapeutic Recreation
edited by Bob Riley

A Recovery Workbook: The Road Back from Substance Abuse
by April K. Neal and Michael J. Taleff

Recreation and Leisure: Issues in an Era of Change, Third Edition
edited by Thomas Goodale and Peter A. Witt

Recreation Economic Decisions: Comparing Benefits and Costs, Second Edition
by John B. Loomis and Richard G. Walsh

Recreation for Older Adults: Individual and Group Activities
by Judith A. Elliott and Jerold E. Elliott

Recreation Programming and Activities for Older Adults
by Jerold E. Elliott and Judith A. Sorg-Elliott

Reference Manual for Writing Rehabilitation Therapy Treatment Plans
by Penny Hogberg and Mary Johnson

Research in Therapeutic Recreation: Concepts and Methods
edited by Marjorie J. Malkin and Christine Z. Howe

Simple Expressions: Creative and Therapeutic Arts for the Elderly in Long-Term Care Facilities
by Vicki Parsons

A Social History of Leisure Since 1600
by Gary Cross

A Social Psychology of Leisure
by Roger C. Mannell and Douglas A. Kleiber

Special Events and Festivals: How to Organize, Plan, and Implement
by Angie Prosser and Ashli Rutledge

Steps to Successful Programming: A Student Handbook to Accompany Programming for Parks, Recreation, and Leisure Services
by Donald G. DeGraaf, Debra J. Jordan, and Kathy H. DeGraaf

Stretch Your Mind and Body: Tai Chi as an Adaptive Activity
by Duane A. Crider and William R. Klinger

Therapeutic Activity Intervention with the Elderly: Foundations and Practices
by Barbara A. Hawkins, Marti E. May, and Nancy Brattain Rogers

Therapeutic Recreation and the Nature of Disabilities
by Kenneth E. Mobily and Richard D. MacNeil

Therapeutic Recreation: Cases and Exercises, Second Edition
by Barbara C. Wilhite and M. Jean Keller

Therapeutic Recreation in Health Promotion and Rehabilitation
by John Shank and Catherine Coyle

Therapeutic Recreation in the Nursing Home
by Linda Buettner and Shelley L. Martin

Therapeutic Recreation Protocol for Treatment of Substance Addictions
by Rozanne W. Faulkner

Tourism and Society: A Guide to Problems and Issues
by Robert W. Wyllie

A Training Manual for Americans with Disabilities Act Compliance in Parks and Recreation Settings
by Carol Stensrud

Venture Publishing, Inc.
1999 Cato Avenue
State College, PA 16801
Phone: (814) 234–4561
Fax: (814) 234–1651